Developing Person-centred Practice

Developing Person-centred Practice

A Practical Approach to Quality Healthcare

Jaqui Hewitt-Taylor

First published 2015 by
PALGRAVE

Palgrave in the UK is an imprint of Macmillan Publishers Limited, registered in England, company number 785998, of 4 Crinan Street, London N1 9XW.

Palgrave Macmillan in the US is a division of St Martin's Press LLC, 175 Fifth Avenue, New York, NY 10010.

Palgrave is a global imprint of the above companies and is represented throughout the world.

Palgrave® and Macmillan® are registered trademarks in the United States, the United Kingdom, Europe and other countries.

ISBN: 978–1–137–39978–6

This book is printed on paper suitable for recycling and made from fully managed and sustained forest sources. Logging, pulping and manufacturing processes are expected to conform to the environmental regulations of the country of origin.

A catalogue record for this book is available from the British Library.

A catalog record for this book is available from the Library of Congress.

Typeset by Aardvark Editorial Limited, Metfield, Suffolk.

Printed in China.

To my nine-year-old son John, who finds Lego and
machines easier to understand than people,
except for his best friend Huxley

Contents

Introducing Person-centred Care and Practice Development 1

Developing person-centred care

In order for patients to receive good quality healthcare, practice has to evolve in light of the latest health-related knowledge, developments in other fields and changes in society. To this end, in the UK, the Nursing and Midwifery Council (NMC 2008), the Health and Care Professions Council (HCPC 2012) and the General Medical Council (GMC 2013) require practitioners to engage in lifelong learning and continually develop their competence and performance.

As well as this requirement for practice to develop, for care to be deemed to be of good quality, it is generally considered necessary for it to be person centred (Innes et al. 2006, RCN 2009, van den Pol-Grevelink et al. 2012). This view is supported by a number of government policies and professional principles (Scottish Government 2009, Manley et al. 2011, DH 2012, 2013, State Government of Victoria 2012). The recommendations from the UK Francis Report (Francis 2013) also place person-centredness as the cornerstone of high-quality care. Good quality healthcare is therefore usually regarded as that which, in addition to being technically proficient, focuses on the person for whom care is being provided, rather than on processes or procedures. As a result, developing high-quality care is often linked with developing person-centred practice.

The term 'developing practice' does not, however, necessarily refer to developing person-centred practice. It can be used to describe many approaches to improving care provision, ranging from developing a new protocol for a specific procedure, through to altering the way in which practitioners perceive and interact with the people they care for (King and Kelly 2011). All these can be very valuable. Using outdated protocols may be detrimental to the care of individual patients and the smooth and efficient running of organizations as a whole, which in turn impacts on the health and wellbeing of many patients.

However, developing an improved protocol or procedure will usually primarily affect the particular element of care that it relates to, and is unlikely to alter the principles that guide practitioners' work. For instance, a new protocol for administering intravenous drugs may greatly improve the efficiency of drug administration and reduce the risk of infection for a large number of patients. This is certainly a good thing, but it will primarily affect the aspects of patients' health associated with intravenous drug administration, although it may have additional associated benefits such as shorter stays for patients and reduced workload for staff. Developments that focus on enabling staff to become more person centred in their approach to care have much less specific, but often wider reaching, outcomes for staff as well as patients. Person-centred practice development means that the key question is not so much: 'Has anything improved?' but: 'Is the way we work now more person centred than it was?' This is the approach to developing practice that this book discusses.

Person-centredness

Person-centredness is discussed in detail in Chapter 2, but essentially means that people are the focus of events. Person-centred care requires people's individuality, humanity, dignity and rights to be recognized, respected and consistently acted on throughout each care encounter (McCormack et al. 2009). It happens when practitioners concentrate their attention on the person they are caring for, how they view the world and what matters to them, rather than on the tasks or procedures that need to be performed.

While person-centred practice moves the focus of care from tasks or processes to the individual to whom care is provided, it still requires practitioners to be knowledgeable, competent and confident in the practical tasks they undertake. Far from devaluing such skills and knowledge, person-centred practice development recognizes the importance of practitioners being knowledgeable, skilled and confident enough to engage with the people they are caring for, and to think flexibly about how best to meet their individual needs.

Working in a person-centred way almost certainly improves the quality of the care from the perspective of those receiving it. There is also a suggestion that it enhances job satisfaction for those providing care (van den Pol-Grevelink et al. 2012). Nonetheless, developing person-centred practice and working in this way day to day is not easy. Few practitioners intentionally aim to work in a non-person-centred way, but many individuals and organizations find it difficult to achieve, for a variety of reasons. These reasons include resources, structures and organizational policies, but also individual values and priorities and workplace cultures.

Practice pointer 1.1

- Person-centredness focuses on seeing people as individuals whose humanity, dignity and rights are important.
- Person-centred care means that care is provided in a way that prioritizes viewing the people who are currently patients in this way.

Resources and structures

Practice not being person centred, or not developing in this way, is often attributed to a lack of resources, both human and material. Resources undoubtedly affect the nature and quality of care provision and how it can develop (Carradice and Round 2009, King and Kelly 2011). If the resources needed to develop and provide person-centred care cannot be secured, it will be difficult to achieve this. Conversely, if adequate resources do exist, it is likely to be easier to deliver person-centred care, and to persuade people to join in ventures aimed at this goal. Resources will not, of themselves, be enough to ensure the development and maintenance of person-centred care, but their absence will affect its achievement.

Staffing issues are recognized as a key factor in the quality of care (CQC 2012). Poor staffing levels make the practicalities of developing practice challenging and tend to have a negative impact on morale, which in turn reduces people's motivation to develop practice (Moody and Pesut 2006). However, as well as numbers of staff, the mix of skills those staff have is important. For example, in nursing, 'skill mix' usually refers to the number of registered nurses (RNs) compared to healthcare assistants (HCAs) in a given situation, with a suggestion that a higher ratio of RNs to HCAs improves care (McCormack and McCance 2010). Besides having an effect on direct day-to-day care, the skill mix of staff is likely to influence how much time and effort can be devoted to practice development initiatives (King and Kelly 2011). As Chapter 4 will discuss, the process of developing person-centred practice focuses on taking time to engage in careful and critical reflective thinking and dialogue. For this to be achievable, staffing numbers and skill mix need to be adequate (Carradice and Round 2009, Hemingway and Cowdell 2009).

In addition to human and material resources, the structures and priorities within organizations influence the development and delivery of person-centred care (McCormack et al. 2007). Structures include practical systems and the way in which workload and staff are allocated. These affect the ease with which developments in practice can be implemented, and influence people's motivation, morale and inclination to give high-quality care and spend time in developing practice. To support the development of person-centred care, organizations therefore need to go beyond stating that it is desirable, to having structures in place that enable and encourage this to happen (McGeehan et al. 2009).

Nonetheless, even where funding, resources and staffing are adequate, or even good, and the structures in place support person-centred care, individual practitioners have to want to work in this way in order for it to become a reality (Jordan 2009).

Individual values, beliefs and priorities

It is impossible for person-centred care to develop unless practitioners subscribe to this ethos and are committed to making it happen. Working in a person-centred way is not something that can be required or imposed by others. Individuals have to be genuinely convinced of its importance, in principle and in terms of it being enough of a priority to devote time and energy to achieving in their own day-to-day practice. For this reason, as Chapter 4 discusses, the process of developing person-centred practice focuses on practitioners engaging in reflection and dialogue, in which they can explore their values, priorities and how they view their work, workplace and those they care for. The intention is for individuals and groups to have the opportunity to critically and honestly question what is important to them, how they want to practise and what enables and inhibits this becoming a reality.

Unless individuals want, and are able, to provide person-centred care, organizations will be unable to create a culture in which this is the norm. Equally, though, unless organizations nurture cultures in which person-centred care can be provided, individual practitioners will struggle to achieve this. The Care Quality Commission (CQC 2012) identifies that poor quality care is generally associated with cultures in which this is the norm, rather than the deliberate actions of individual practitioners. Workplace cultures, which include the structures, priorities, values, beliefs and ways of working of individuals and groups, are therefore key determinants of whether or not person-centred care can be achieved and sustained (McCormack and McCance 2010).

Practice pointer 1.2

Developing person-centred care requires:

- adequate resources and staffing levels
- structures and systems that support person-centred care
- individuals and teams who want this to happen.

Workplace cultures

There is not complete consensus about what organizational or workplace culture means (Scott et al. 2003, Kirkley et al. 2011). However, it is generally thought to include the social environment, relationships, attitudes to work, expected behaviours, rituals, beliefs, values, rules (written and unwritten) and history of a workplace or organization (Cameron and Green 2009, Parkin 2009, McCormack and McCance 2010, Kirkley et al. 2011). These work together to influence the behaviour of individuals and groups and impact on most aspects of workplace life, such as how work is carried out, how and by whom decisions are made, how rewards (both formal and informal) are allocated, and how people are treated (McCormack and McCance 2010).

Culture is not static, but constantly evolves through ongoing, usually informal and often subconscious negotiations between the people who make up that culture (Jordan 2009). Thus, a person-centred culture may be eroded, but equally a culture that is not particularly person centred can become person centred. There may also be a difference between the espoused values of a culture and what happens in reality (McCormack and McCance 2010). For example, a ward may, in theory, subscribe to the values of person-centredness, but for a number of reasons, the day-to-day reality of practice may be very different.

A workplace culture is often seen as the mode of operating that the people in a particular work setting adhere to. Although not everyone in a workplace will share the same opinions, values or beliefs, the dominant culture tends to influence everyone's beliefs, values and behaviour to some extent. For example, a newly qualified practitioner, taking up their first job, is likely to want to fit in and be liked in their workplace. To do so, they may well feel the need to embrace the behaviours, values and priorities of the group they wish, or need, to become a part of (Thompson et al. 2006). If the culture in which they find themselves values, prioritizes and rewards person-centred working, the newcomer will feel uncomfortable and find it difficult to fit in if they do not also adopt, or at least appear to adopt, these values and behaviours. Thus, culture can positively influence the way in which practitioners learn to work. Conversely, if a practitioner aspires to work in a person-centred way, but finds themselves in a culture where the priority is meeting targets and completing tasks, they may find it hard to be accepted if they seek to practise in accordance with their ideals. If they remain in this workplace, the dominant culture is likely, over time, to erode their commitment to being person centred in their work. To be able to practise person-centred care, individuals therefore need to feel that this is culturally acceptable and be confident that they will not be criticized, judged harshly, ridiculed or ostracized for choosing to work in this way.

While workplace cultures are created by a combination of the individual people who work in a particular setting, they are also affected by the wider organization to which that setting belongs. Although individual practitioners may be highly motivated to work in a person-centred way, Chin and Hamer (2006) identify the importance of influential peers and leaders modelling this throughout the organization within which they work. In order for the care provided to individual patients to be person centred, organizations need this to be role modelled and seen as truly prized and celebrated by those in positions of influence or authority.

Healthcare increasingly requires professions and disciplines to work together (RCN/RCP 2006, Atwal and Jones 2007, Macphee and Suryaprakash 2012). Each team, and the professions or disciplines which are a part of, or work with, that team, is likely to have their own, potentially differing cultures, which affect how they work (Kirkley et al. 2011). As a result, the culture of care in any healthcare team or organization is likely to be influenced by the prevailing culture of a number of disciplines or professions (Wilson et al. 2006). The process of developing a culture of person-centred care is, therefore, an endeavour that needs to include individuals, teams and organizations, and cross disciplinary boundaries. To achieve this, a systematic approach, such as that encountered in practice development methodology, is often useful.

Practice pointer 1.3

- Workplace cultures are critical to whether or not person-centred care is achieved.
- Workplace cultures are influenced by the values, beliefs, priorities and history of individuals, groups, teams, professions, disciplines and organizations.

Practice development methodology

Practice development methodology, discussed in Chapter 2, centres on the processes that will assist people and workplaces to develop person-centred practice (McCormack et al. 2009). While its person-centred ethos means that it focuses on individuals, it also sees each person as part of their wider social environment, and recognizes that development of the individual practitioner cannot be fully achieved without considering the social and cultural situation within which they work.

Practice development methodology therefore acknowledges that achieving real and lasting developments in practice requires attention to be given to matters that lie within the organization, the individual and the combination of the individual and the corporate that creates organizational culture (McCormack 2008). To achieve this, it uses a systematic and rigorous approach to developing person-centred practice (McCormack 2008).

A guide to the book

This book aims to systematically describe how the process of developing person-centred practice can be approached. The early chapters discuss some of the concepts that underpin practice development methodology and their practical application. These are followed by chapters that discuss more discrete, specific aspects of the development of person-centred practice.

The complexity of developing person-centred practice means that each aspect of it requires individual, group, cultural, social and organizational factors to be considered. In order to address these interrelated elements, every chapter is drawn around a case study.

Each chapter begins with an overview that outlines its contents, and is interspersed with summaries of key points and activities that invite the reader to consider the application of what is being presented to their own practice. A worked example is provided at the end of every chapter, to draw these activities together. All the chapters are also appended by a short section in which web-based resources related to their contents are suggested, to provide a convenient means for the reader to access further information about the key subjects covered.

In the absence of consensus on the best terminology for the people to whom healthcare is provided, the term 'patient' is generally used in this book. However, the person referred to as a patient is an individual human being, who could be you or me.

Chapter 2 introduces the theoretical basis of practice development methodology. This includes its core concept of person-centredness and the underpinnings of critical social theory and critical realism. The chapter concludes by focusing on how emancipation and transformation of practitioners is needed to enable them to become critically creative and develop innovative approaches to care.

Chapter 3 explores in detail the central concept of practice development methodology, person-centredness. This includes discussions of personhood, citizenship, what person-centredness is, and what this means in terms of providing care that is person centred. The chapter addresses the importance of staff as well as patients being seen as people, and why person-centredness is considered to be beneficial, enhance care and working environments. It also highlights what may be needed to achieve person-centred care, in terms of individuals, groups and organizations.

Chapter 4 introduces some of the ways in which a culture of person-centred practice development may be initiated, achieved and sustained. It starts by discussing the need to create a culture of learning, with person-centredness at its core, and then explores approaches to achieving this. These include using the principles of appreciative inquiry, active learning techniques and developing the skills of critical reflection and day-to-day reflexivity. These strands of discussions are brought together to highlight their places in developing a culture in which learning processes are used to free practitioners to be creative and innovative in developing practice.

Person-centred practice development places patients as key, central players in developments. Chapter 5 discusses how meaningful practice development partnerships with patients can be achieved. This includes the purpose of involving patients, who to involve, how to involve people, and the preparation and support that organizations, teams and individuals may need for working in partnership to develop practice.

Chapter 6 discusses the types of information that can be used to inform person-centred practice development. In keeping with the philosophical underpinnings of practice development methodology, it begins by highlighting the importance of personal and tacit knowledge and individual perceptions of what constitutes reality. This is followed by a discussion of hierarchies of evidence, and the nature and value of particular forms of evidence, such as research, systematic review, audit, evaluation, guidelines, case reports and expert opinion. The chapter ends by emphasizing the need to collate the available evidence from across sources to provide a composite picture of what is known and how it might apply to particular practice situations.

Practice development methodology is concerned with ways of thinking and viewing practice rather than changing discrete elements of care. However, understanding the principles of managing change can be useful in engaging individuals and groups in this process. Chapter 7 explores the management of change and its application to developing person-centred practice. In line with the principles of practice development methodology, this discussion focuses primarily on the people factors involved and what will encourage or inhibit individuals and groups from participating in person-centred practice development.

Chapter 8 discusses the importance of leadership in the development of person-centred practice. It begins by distinguishing leadership and management and highlighting the role and function of a leader or leaders in practice development. It then considers approaches to leadership that are compatible with the ethos of person-centred practice, including transformational and authentic leadership. The chapter concludes by discussing the importance of leadership development and succession planning in creating and sustaining a culture of person-centred practice.

Evaluation is a key aspect of any development in practice, and Chapter 9 is concerned with the evaluation of person-centred practice development. It begins by highlighting the need to adopt an approach to evaluation that is congruent with practice development methodology, and then considers the specifics of designing an evaluation that captures the process as well as outcomes of developing person-centred practice. This discussion includes what to evaluate, methods that can be used to evaluate, when to evaluate, who to involve in the evaluation, how evaluative information can be analysed, and the ethical issues involved in evaluation.

Practice development is not just about developing areas where practice is considered poor, but about maintaining and sustaining good practice and making it even better. Chapter 10 discusses the importance of sustaining a culture of person-centred practice development after the initial impetus for innovation is gone and how this may be achieved.

Chapter 11 identifies the importance of the new knowledge that developing person-centred practice generates, and the value of, and possible approaches to, sharing this knowledge. These include local, national and international dissemination through publications, conference presentations and networking opportunities.

Finally, the Endpoints chapter concludes the book by drawing together the ideas presented in the preceding chapters.

2 Practice Development: A Person-centred Methodology

Chapter overview

- The ethos that underpins practice development methodology is person-centredness.
- Practice development methodology focuses on developing person-centred cultures, rather than changing particular elements of practice.
- The principles of critical social theory and critical realism also inform practice development methodology. These consider how systems, structures, individual and group beliefs, values, norms and perceptions of reality contribute to what people do and their level of empowerment.
- The tools that practice development methodology uses are those that enable practitioners to think about what informs and directs their practice. Its intention is to enable individuals and teams to creatively explore options and opportunities to develop person-centred care.

Zayneb has recently been appointed as the ward manager of an acute medical admissions ward. The ward has a team of well-established staff, and things appear to run very efficiently and meet the required targets. The care provided is generally effective and professional, with few errors, omissions or delays. However, Zayneb does not think that it always matches the person-centred ethos that the ward is described as subscribing to and feels that care is often somewhat mechanistic, or task focused. She has been considering how best to address this, and has come across practice development methodology, as described by McCormack et al. (2009), which seems to be the sort of thing she is looking for.

Practice development methodology

The term 'practice development' has been linked to various approaches to altering the way in which care is provided, ranging from changing specific aspects of practice, to transforming workplaces cultures (King and Kelly 2011). The approach that Zayneb has come across describes a methodology that can be used to alter workplace cultures, rather than to change isolated elements of practice (McCormack et al. 2013).

Practice pointer 2.1

Practice development methodology focuses on developing workplace cultures, rather than changing discrete elements of practice.

The term 'methodology' is often used in research, and refers to the values, assumptions and theoretical concepts that underpin and inform a study. These provide the basis for deciding what approaches or tools should be used to gather and analyse information (Clough and Nutbrown 2012). In practice development, the methodology used clarifies the values, assumptions and theoretical concepts that underpin and inform the activities that are undertaken in order to develop practice (Manley and McCormack 2004). Research methodology provides a framework for systematically gathering and analysing information (Kumar 2008). In the same way, the methodology used in practice development should provide the basis for a rigorous and systematic approach to developing practice (Manley and McCormack 2004, Shaw 2013).

The underpinning ethos of practice development methodology is person-centredness (McCormack et al. 2009). Everything done in its name should, therefore, be designed to enhance the person-centredness of care provision. Zayneb's opinion is that the work her team carries out is generally well organized and technically sound. However, she senses that meeting the particular needs or concerns of individuals is not a core aspect of care provision. Thus, practice development methodology seems to her to be an ideal way to try to address what she thinks is lacking in her workplace.

Practice pointer 2.2

The methodology used in practice development should:

- clarify the values and theoretical concepts that underpin the activities undertaken
- provide a framework for rigorously and systematically developing practice.

A person-centred ethos

Person-centredness is discussed in more detail in Chapter 3, but practice development being person centred means that practice should be developed in a way that focuses on people and their particular and individual characteristics and needs (McCormack et al. 2009). This separates practice development methodology from the development of discrete elements of practice (such as altering the way a procedure is carried out, or introducing a new protocol), change management, or service improvement (King and Kelly 2011). In practice development methodology, the goal of whatever is done is to enhance the person-centredness of care provision. Any actions taken need to be consistent with this, and the person or persons to whom care is provided, not the procedures involved, are the central concern.

Activity 2.1

Think about developments or changes that have taken place in your workplace in recent months. What approach to developing practice did they use?

Zayneb has identified several processes and procedures on her ward that could be changed to try to increase the person-centredness of care. These include the approach to gathering information when patients are admitted to the ward and how the transfer of patients to other wards is managed. However, because it is the ethos within which work is carried out, rather than particular tasks, that makes her feel uncomfortable at times, practice development methodology appeals to her. She also thinks that if the whole approach to practice on the ward becomes more person centred, people will naturally seek to alter particular aspects of the way they work, rather than her suggesting piecemeal innovations that do not address the core issue. Zayneb's opinion is that the way in which people are assessed on admission might be improved, to include more of a focus on their priorities, values, concerns and life out of hospital. Nonetheless, while improving the personalization of admission processes and documentation might encourage a greater understanding of each individual's needs, she can see some limitations in focusing on this. For it to be meaningful, the assessment would need to happen in a culture where a core value of all care provision was person-centredness. Otherwise, any additional information-gathering activities carried out on admission might be meaningless, with information recorded but not used. It would also be unlikely to be sustained, as the cultural ethos required to achieve this would not have changed. If, on the other hand, the ward develops a more person-centred work ethos, a natural result is likely to be that staff will see the value of gaining more personalized information about the people they are admitting and will use this information meaningfully.

Activity 2.2

How far do you think the culture of your workplace fits a person-centred ethos?

Practice development methodology aims to develop a culture where honouring the individuality and humanity of those receiving care is highly valued. However, because it focuses on people, it also sees the humanity and individuality of those providing care as vital aspects of developing practice (McCormack and McCance 2006, Manley and McCormack 2008). It therefore seeks to develop practice by exploring how the views, beliefs, values and priorities of the people providing care shape current provision, and to use this knowledge to explore how person-centred care might be initiated or developed further. It also recognizes that individuals may, for a variety of personal, contextual, social and historical reasons, not feel able to alter the way they work. So, a key part of practice development methodology is unpicking how individual, team, professional and organizational structures, beliefs, values, priorities, experiences, history, culture and perceptions influence the achievement of person-centred practice. As a result, the tools that are used primarily aim to enable practitioners to think about what informs and directs their practice (McCormack 2008). Zayneb believes that these approaches will be important in her quest to develop practice on her ward. She is fairly confident that most of the staff want to provide good care and, in theory, subscribe to the ideal of person-centredness. What will be more challenging will be to work with them on exploring how they can make this a day-to-day reality, permeating all aspects of their work.

While Zayneb likes the idea of developing person-centred practice, she recognizes that in order to achieve this, what has contributed to the current status quo and what might need to happen for this to change require consideration. Practice development methodology seems to her to be useful in this respect, as it is informed by theories, such as critical social theory and critical realism. These explore how systems, structures, individual and group beliefs, values, norms and perceptions of reality contribute to what people do, and emphasize the need for individuals and groups to be empowered to transform how they work (Parlour and McCormack 2012).

Practice pointer 2.3

Practice development methodology focuses on how individual, group, professional and organizational views, beliefs, values, priorities, structures, cultures and history influence the achievement of person-centred practice.

Critical social theory

Critical social theory seeks to understand phenomena by exploring the context in which they occur. This includes where something happens, who is involved, and how the knowledge, values and power that individuals and groups have affect it (Freeman and Vasconcelos 2010, Bevan et al. 2012, Lapum et al. 2012). Critical social theory would therefore view all the elements of the practice environment, including where events occur, who is involved in them, and the individual and group beliefs, values and power equations that exist, as influencing every aspect of care.

The principles of critical social theory would suggest that whether the process of admitting people to Zayneb's ward is carried out in a person-centred way depends on:

- the beliefs and values that the person carrying out the admission holds
- what they see as the priorities of the admission process
- what the ward team as a whole views as the priorities of care
- how these relate to the competing calls on their time
- the pressures on the individual at the time of the admission
- what they perceive others think about what they are doing
- the level of influence others have on them
- their knowledge about admission processes
- the structures in place that affect the admission process.

In order to develop person-centred admission practice, more than discrete aspects of the process of admission, for example the questions that are asked, would need to be addressed. This would include thinking about how individuals' beliefs, values and priorities, and the prevailing beliefs, values and priorities on the ward interlink with organizational structures and competing demands to result in what is currently the accepted approach to admitting patients to the ward.

To achieve this understanding, critical social theory identifies the need to have conversations that go beyond the immediate concerns that individuals may have, or state that they have, about the phenomena of interest. This type of discourse includes exploring and appraising people's principles, beliefs, values and priorities related to the matter in question, and what enables or hinders them in achieving what they would ideally like to do (Freeman and Vasconcelos 2010). Zayneb thinks that this would be a good way for her to approach developing practice on her ward. Instead of discussing adjusting particular aspects of care, she wants to explore people's views about their work and workplace, uncover what their priorities are and what they want to achieve, and consider what contributes to or prevents them from working in the way they want to. In order to achieve this, as Chapter 4 will discuss, practice development methodology uses tools such as critical reflection to enable individuals and groups to think about what drives and influences their work, whether they are satisfied with the way things are, and what might help them to develop their practice.

As well as considering the current events that influence situations, critical social theory sees it as vital to appreciate how a group, team or organization's structure and history, and the history of those within it, shape what it is today (Freeman and Vasconcelos 2010). For Zayneb, this would mean looking at how the history, structure and functions of the organization, the professions within this, the ward itself and the histories of the individual people working on the ward inhibit or facilitate person-centred working. This might include power issues, permitted and perceived levels of autonomy or authority and individuals' histories and experiences in previous workplaces. As a newcomer, it may be particularly helpful for Zayneb to understand why her team functions in the way it does, but she also thinks that it will be valuable for the established ward team to explore and challenge why they see things as they do, and work in particular ways.

Activity 2.3

Think about how your values affect your work. How are these values influenced by your colleagues' values?

Practice pointer 2.4

Critical social theory seeks to understand phenomena by exploring:

- the context in which the phenomenon occurs
- the principles, beliefs, values and priorities of the individuals involved
- the power that individuals and groups hold or are perceived to hold.

Empowerment

While all the aspects of what has created the current status quo of a workplace are considered important, the central tenet of critical social theory is empowerment (Bevan et al. 2012). It holds that power and oppression significantly shape the behaviour of individuals and groups, and sees it as necessary to overcome all forms of oppression in order to facilitate personal and group development. Individuals or groups who are, or perceive themselves to be, lacking power or in vulnerable positions will probably not feel able to attempt to alter how things are (Lapum et al. 2012). They are unlikely to think that others will listen to their ideas or consider them worthy of action, and may therefore see no reason to share their opinions or attempt to develop practice. People may also find it difficult to take responsibility for what happens in their workplace if they view themselves as powerless to influence this. In addition, those who are themselves oppressed, or feel devalued, are not usually well placed to value and seek to empower others.

In order to develop practice, critical social theory sees it as vital to explore what prevents people from having, or perceiving themselves to have, the power to act as they might wish to. This need for staff to feel empowered in order to effect innovations in practice has resonance with current health policy in the UK, as well as practice development methodology (King and Kelly 2011), and Zayneb considers it an important issue in her workplace. She has, on two or three occasions, heard nurses on her ward asking colleagues about doing things slightly differently and being told that it 'wouldn't go down well'. When she has intervened to ask who would object, the answer has not always been clear. On one occasion, a medical consultant's preferences were cited and on another she was advised that: 'I don't think it'd go down well if the matrons got to hear.' However, when Zayneb suggested the idea to the unit matron, no objections were raised. This has led Zayneb to consider what power issues exist, or are perceived to exist, within the organization, but also on the ward itself, which inhibit staff from developing their practice.

Activity 2.4

Consider how the history, culture, structure, functions and power equations of the team you work in influence care provision.

Zayneb's ward is a busy acute admissions ward, where the nurses she manages work with members of many other disciplines and teams. Fielding et al. (2008) suggest that nurses have, historically, been viewed as an oppressed group, lacking in power in a health system where medicine and its values have dominated. In addition, McCormack and McCance (2010) identify that the hierarchical power structures traditionally held in nursing itself have affected the culture in which nurses practise. Although power relationships between nursing and other professions, and within nursing, may have changed, the profession's history is still likely to influence how nurses perceive themselves and how they see power as working. The way the nurses on Zayneb's ward view themselves in relation to the other professions they work with, and the structure of their own profession, may affect the way they provide and prioritize care. It may also influence their perceptions of their ability to change things and the people whose permission or approval they consider they need in order to develop practice, even in areas that fall within a predominantly nursing domain.

Nonetheless, although looking at formal structures and hierarchical power equations is important, it is useful to remember that horizontal as well as vertical power exists and can strongly influence practice (McCormack and McCance 2010). Informal power and influence among peers may be as strong, and even stronger, and more empowering or disempowering than that based on formal positions (McCormack and McCance 2010). Zayneb thinks that this will be an important part of exploring person-centred practice on her ward, as she has noticed that it is not always the more senior nurses who appear to hold the most influence. She has identified that the opinion of one of the HCAs is frequently sought, and acted on, by other staff. It seems that she and one of the RNs who is popular, but not especially senior, will be key influences in any developments, because of the informal power and influence they hold. The discussions she has been involved in about suggestions to change aspects of practice have also made her wonder whether the reasons cited for these being problematic really represent a perception that the medical staff or matrons will object. She has a suspicion that the people who raised these difficulties opposed the suggested changes themselves, but used the anticipated responses of others within the perceived hierarchy as a more convenient or convincing argument than their own objections.

Practice pointer 2.5

Critical social theory sees all forms of power and oppression, and people's perceptions of these, as significantly shaping events and people's perceptions of these events.

Critical social theory sees the views and perceptions of everyone involved in a situation as important (Freeman and Vasconcelos 2010). As such, patients' priorities, values, beliefs, history and perceptions of personal and joint power are a crucial part of developing practice. Unless these are known, developments in care cannot be truly person centred, as the most vital people's priorities will not be represented. Chapter 3 discusses person-centredness in more detail, and Chapter 5 explores how patients can be meaningfully involved in practice development initiatives. However, in terms of critical social theory's emphasis on empowerment, the patients on Zayneb's ward are generally acutely unwell. As such, Zayneb thinks they are likely to be, or perceive themselves to be, vulnerable and lacking in power. This may be a significant contrast to their usual level of autonomy or power. In addition, historically, patients were seen as the passive and subservient recipients of what professionals considered was best for them. Despite attempts to challenge and alter this division of power, it may still influence how patients as well as staff perceive care provision, their place in it, and their ability and right to challenge or question matters (Braye and Preston-Shoot 2005, Higgins et al. 2011).

Zayneb thinks that using practice development methodology, with its focus on person-centredness and underpinning principles of critical social theory, is what she wants for her ward. However, she is also aware that she may need to justify, to herself and others, why she is not primarily focusing on improving particular aspects of practice. One element of critical social theory that Zayneb has found useful in understanding and planning an explanation of this is the work of Habermas (1971), which outlines three types of interest or knowledge.

Three types of knowledge

Habermas, one of the theorists whose work contributes to critical social theory, identified three different types of interest or knowledge: technical, practical and emancipatory. These are all interlinked and necessary to effect meaningful understanding of situations and lasting changes in how things are done (Habermas 1971).

Technical interest

Technical interest, as the name suggests, concerns technical knowledge and skills. Habermas (1971) suggests that such knowledge serves a valuable purpose, but is not the only legitimate type of knowledge. In healthcare, technical and practical processes need to be understood and carried out correctly, so this kind of knowledge is essential. Changing practice in a way that focuses on this sort of knowledge also has clear benefits, in that a specific aspect of care provision is improved. However, it may not lead to sustainable change, or change outside the particular procedure or process involved (Sanders et al. 2013). Habermas (1971) specifically identifies that technical knowledge alone is not enough to understand human motivation and actions. Zayneb thinks that this is a key issue for her team, because although technical knowledge is clearly a vital part of the work on her ward, she wants to focus on what people see as important in care situations and why they act as they do. A technical or procedural change in how admissions or transfers to other wards are conducted might improve some elements of care. However, for people to carry out person-centred care, every aspect of their work, not just a particular part of it, will need to be underpinned by this ethos. In addition, those concerned will have to see this as important and worthy of making the effort to achieve.

In approaches that focus primarily on developing technical aspects of practice, the person leading the development is perceived as the expert, who is in charge of the innovation, knows what has to be done, how it should be done and the criteria for success (Manley and McCormack 2003). This is sometimes necessary, for example when something in practice is unsafe and requires prompt action, without a great deal of time for discussion or reflection. However, one of the difficulties with this approach is that it can become a part of quick fixes and behaviourally driven solutions to problems or challenges. These may address particular issues, but do not change the way individuals or teams see their work, and, if used in isolation, often fail to address the underlying problems that created a need for solutions (McCormack 2008). In addition, Zayneb does not want to be seen to be instigating change for the sake of change, or in order to stamp her authority on her new team. Instead, her aim is to create a culture in which staff all take a lead in developments, and value and own the way in which they work. Rather than a top-down approach to change, with alterations in practice imposed by those who manage services, Zayneb wants to develop a culture in which developments in practice are designed and owned by frontline staff – a bottom-up approach (Manley and McCormack 2003). Her goal is to develop a team who feel able and willing to question their own practice and that of others, and a culture where innovation is sustained and continued.

At the same time, Zayneb thinks that it is important that the people who work on the ward are competent and feel confident in the technical aspects of the care they provide. Otherwise, they are unlikely to be able to move beyond concerns about particular tasks or procedures and focus on the people they are caring for and their individual circumstances, values, priorities and needs.

Practical interest

The second type of interest identified by Habermas (1971) is practical interest, which concerns how others see their world. This creates knowledge and understanding that goes beyond what should, technically, work well, to include what things may mean for other people, how this will affect what they are prepared to engage with, and what works or does not. Practical knowledge includes:

- an understanding of how individuals would be likely to view something
- how it would fit into their worldview
- what threats and opportunities it would create or be perceived to create for them
- whether it would be important or a priority for them
- whether they would be likely to embrace or participate in it.

As Chapter 7 will explore, these are key issues in managing any change in practice, including change aimed at achieving a more person-centred way of working. It is the type of knowledge that is generally gained through spending time with people and groups, and in dialogue with them, in order to understand them, their beliefs, values and interpretations of situations. Habermas's (1971) work emphasizes that everyone is likely to have slightly different values, priorities and perceptions, all of which affect what they do. Thus, his work places seeing people as individuals and exploring how they perceive the world as key elements of understanding situations and effecting lasting change.

As well as considering how staff perceive their work and workplace, gaining practical knowledge in the context of developing person-centred care includes considering how patients see their world and their experiences of healthcare. This type of knowledge enables practitioners to think about what the care they provide might mean, or be perceived to mean, by the people who are currently patients. This involves spending time with patients and engaging in meaningful dialogue in which what really matters to them can be explored.

Zayneb can see that in order to understand why the staff on her ward practise as they do, it will be necessary for her to gain practical knowledge of how they view their work and whether developing a more person-centred approach would fit this. This will include:

- what threats and opportunities person-centred care might create or be perceived to create for them
- whether it would be important or a priority for them
- whether they would be likely to embrace the idea.

To glean this information, spending time and engaging in open and nonjudgmental dialogue with them will be necessary. Equally, without staff wanting, and being able, to develop practical knowledge of their patients, they will not be able to care for them in a person-centred way. Thus, to move the ward culture to being more person centred, Zayneb considers that having this type of practical knowledge of staff, but staff also seeing this type of knowledge of patients as important, will be crucial.

Emancipatory interest

The third element of Habermas's (1971) knowledge, emancipatory interest, is concerned with understanding oneself and how the world in which one functions is influenced by social conditions. This relates to knowledge about the things within individuals but also outwith them, which influences their perception of themselves, their present and past experiences and their level of empowerment (Bevan et al. 2012).

In terms of developing person-centred practice, this includes the things within individual practitioners and in their workplace that enable or prevent them from feeling that they can work in a person-centred way. Zayneb is interested in identifying what, in the organization as a whole and the ward itself, her colleagues think enables or prevents them from working in a person-centred way. She also wants to explore what influences patients' expectations and what they feel they can ask for in care. In addition, she thinks that enabling individual practitioners to consider what makes them feel able or unable to develop the way they work, and what influences this, will be a key part of developing person-centred care.

While Zayneb has focused on how she can work with her staff to develop more person-centred care, her perceptions are also an important part of the equation. This includes her perceptions of what staff currently do, what she thinks enables and detracts from them providing person-centred care, and what influences her thinking. She is working on the basis that she feels that care on the ward could be more person centred, and that the ward team are in a position to change their practice in this respect. However, she has to question what her perceptions are fuelled by, what motivates her to think in this way, and how her perceptions compare to those of other key players, including patients. In addition, she needs to consider how her own, as well as other people's, motivations and actions are influenced by the wider social and organizational structures they work within.

Zayneb thinks that using a combination of emancipatory, practical and technical knowledge will enable her to work with her team towards exploring whether they can develop practice so that it becomes more person centred. Crucially, it will also enable her to consider her own role, influences and motivations in this. Any practice development activity is inevitably enmeshed in a complex mix of the individuals concerned, the way in which individuals contribute to groups, and how groups function within wider organizations.

One of the things Zayneb finds attractive in practice development methodology is that it acknowledges this complexity. Another element of the theory underpinning practice development methodology that she finds useful in articulating its nature is the influence of critical realism.

Practice pointer 2.6

Habermas's (1971) three types of knowledge or interest are technical, practical and emancipatory.

Activity 2.5

Think about the different types of knowledge you use in practice. How do they fit into Habermas's categories of technical, practical and emancipatory knowledge?

Critical realism

Critical realism essentially deals with reality, how it is perceived, and how this affects people's decisions and actions. It begins by questioning what exists, or is thought to exist, and then moves on to question how we know (or think we know) that this exists (Bergin et al. 2008). While critical realism assumes that an objective reality does exist, it also identifies that there are many different perceptions of what is real. In addition, it notes that the language used to describe even the most objective reality, the meaning it has for people and the social context in which it exists influence how it is perceived (Oliver 2012). Critical realism considers it almost impossible for people to completely step outside their own perspectives and therefore sees a gap between objective reality and individual perceptions or descriptions of this as virtually inevitable.

Zayneb believes that this appreciation that people genuinely perceive things differently will help her to understand her own and her colleagues' perspectives, and why each person feels it best, or necessary, to practise in certain ways. She also realizes that patients' individual perceptions influence their views on the quality of care provision. For care to become person centred, acknowledgement of the perceptions of all the people involved, including patients and practitioners, needs to be a part of the complex 'reality' of practice.

Critical realism sees the world operating as a complex multidimensional open system (Harwood and Clark 2012, Parlour and McCormack 2012). This means that while the many different elements of any given situation are interlinked and interact with each other, these interactions work in different ways in different contexts. Thus, a given action can produce different outcomes on different occasions, even when the same people are involved, because a multitude of nuances of a situation and interpretation of this influence one another (Cruickshank 2012). Zayneb is aware, for example, that while she subscribes in theory to the ethos of person-centredness, the extent to which her practice is person centred can vacillate from day to day. This is influenced by her workload, who she is working with, their views, their influence on her, the patients she is caring for, how confident she feels in meeting their care needs, and whether she is in a good mood that day. It also depends on the priority she affords person-centred care, what she perceives this to mean, and what she thinks people would appreciate in their care. Thus, it is impossible to predict that she will always provide a particular degree of person-centred care, as perceived by everyone concerned. She might on one day, because the ward is well staffed, she is working with a team who enable her to work in this way, has slept well the night before, had a good journey to work, and is caring for patients whose care needs she is confident in meeting. On another occasion, one or more of these variables might change how things are done or perceived by her, her colleagues or the people she is caring for.

Rather than seeking to find approaches that will always work, critical realism looks for conclusions that are dynamic and dependent on the context and variations of a given situation. These conclusions are termed 'outcome patterns', and include not just why an intervention may result in a particular outcome, but what particular aspects of a situation interact, and how they interact, to produce a given outcome (Oliver 2012). Zayneb thinks that this represents some of the challenges involved in developing person-centred practice. Acknowledging the multifactorial nature of reality may enable her to explore with people why intentions to provide person-centred care might not always work, or be perceived to work, in all situations or by all parties.

Practice pointer 2.7

Critical realism posits that:

- an objective reality exists
- there are many different perceptions of what is real
- context, time and other people affect each individual's perception of reality
- a given action can produce different outcomes on different occasions because the circumstances in which it happens are different.

Critical realism, like critical social theory, aims to achieve emancipation of individuals and provides a structure for challenging surface appearances by exploring what generates these and the perceptions of reality that influence them (Oliver 2012). It enables the questions about why everyday events occur and why people feel and act the way they do to be asked. From this, the causes of people being or feeling oppressed and unable to influence their own situation can proceed. For example, critical realism would seek to explore the reasons why a nurse in a particular situation felt unable to practise in a person-centred way, despite wanting to. It looks beyond the individual to corporate causes, such as how teams and organizations perceive reality and how the multiple events and perceptions that exist interact to produce outcomes. Thus, it acknowledges the complex and interrelated causes of situations, and encourages action that goes beyond surface interventions to tackle the deeper roots of issues, key among these being what facilitates, or reduces, empowerment (Oliver 2012). This is what Zayneb thinks is needed for her ward to move towards more person-centred practice. However, she also believes that for person-centred practice to develop, she and her team will need to create a vision of what they want their ward to be like, the kind of care they want to give and how they would ideally like to provide this.

Practice pointer 2.8

By seeking to understand how people perceive things and what influences these perceptions, critical realism provides a structure for people to become empowered to perceive things and therefore act differently.

Critical creativity

The transformation of thinking and emancipation that practice development methodology focuses on should provide an opportunity for people to creatively imagine innovative approaches to practice (Titchen and McMahon 2013). This, alongside a recognition of the value of every person and the contribution they can make, gives teams the opportunity to blend each individual's personal qualities, knowledge, skills, wisdom and imagination to design something unique, which contributes to facilitating person-centred care (Manley et al. 2013a). This should enable practice to develop beyond known options, to people imagining their ideal way of working and striving to achieve something that meets that vision, even if it falls outside the boundaries of standard practice (Shaw 2013).

Practice pointer 2.9

Critical creativity enables individuals and teams to move beyond standard approaches to care and design innovative, person-centred options.

Zayneb likes this aspect of practice development methodology. When she has tentatively suggested modification of the admission process, this has been met with comments about the limitations of the alternative options that are known to exist and why they will not work in the milieu of a busy admissions ward. She thinks that using the critical creativity that practice development methodology facilitates may enable her to work with her team to think beyond these known options and the traditions of what is acceptable in acute care to explore other, more innovative approaches. She sees this as a key aspect of person-centredness for staff and patients, because while patient experiences will be improved, staff will also have the chance to grow, develop and contribute something uniquely theirs to practice (Manley et al. 2013a, Titchen and McMahon 2013).

Activity 2.6

Think about a recent interaction with a patient that you were involved in, and try to unpick all the things, positive and negative, that influenced that interaction.

Practice pointer 2.10

Practice development methodology draws on the principles of critical realism, critical social theory and critical creativity to enable individuals and teams to develop a more person-centred approach to care.

Summary

Practice development methodology holds that person-centred care can be most effectively achieved by enabling practitioners to understand their own priorities, beliefs, values and perceptions of reality, and how these and the structures and systems within which they work contribute to care provision. It creates the opportunity for people to challenge the status quo on an individual and organizational level, and, as a result, to develop creative and imaginative approaches to their work, resulting in more person-centred care (McCormack et al. 2006, Wilson and McCormack 2006).

The processes used to enable practice development of this kind are those that allow people to review, question, explore and transform their perceptions of their work, workplace and practice. These have, as their natural conclusion, a workforce that seeks to constantly question, refine and develop practice, and a culture in which creative innovation is nurtured (Wilson and McCormack 2006). This is what Zayneb wants for her team. It is likely to be a slower process than trying to alter particular aspects of care and will not provide quick fixes for perceived problems. It may also highlight that person-centredness will be difficult to achieve on her ward or is not what people want. However, working in this way will enable Zayneb and her team to identify and own their values and beliefs, and to work realistically from this point, rather than making assumptions about what matters, or should matter, to individuals.

Zayneb's own view, and the ethos of the methodology she wants to use, is that achieving person-centredness is a key goal. However, before taking her plans further, she wants to make sure she has really understood what person-centredness is and means in practice.

Case scenario

Faith works as a community nurse. Her team's caseload includes a high proportion of older people, many of whom need visits for more than one reason and require assistance with daily care as well as particular treatments. Faith thinks that her team generally do a very good job: they try to stay up to date with developments in practice and provide a high standard of care. However, Faith has recently been considering how her team works and whether there is anything that could be done to improve this. This was prompted by a visit she made to Mr Edwards. She had visited Mr Edwards a few times over the past year to administer vitamin B12 injections, remove sutures after a surgical procedure and do dressings when he developed a wound on his leg. On this occasion, she mentioned that her son was studying the Second World War at school. Mr Edwards told her that he had been a gunner on an aircraft in the war, and shared some of his memories with her. Mr Edwards' recollections made Faith wonder how much she missed of who the people she cared for were and the importance of this in her work and interactions with them. It also made her think about what her team as a whole did, how they did it and what they valued in their work.

The developments or changes that have taken place in Faith's workplace recently and the approaches they used to developing practice

Faith thought about the ways in which her team had developed their practice over the past two years. They had developed new approaches to managing leg ulcer dressings, administering medication via long lines, and assessing patient needs. These were important developments and certainly enhanced care. They were, however, developments that addressed particular procedures or processes.

These developments had all come about because of suggestions within the team, not managerial requests or requirements. The team as a whole generally felt able and confident to suggest new ideas to one another, and were receptive to trying new things. However, none of the developments had been concerned with the ethos of care – probably because no one saw this as requiring change, or able to be changed.

How far did Faith think her team's culture fitted a person-centred ethos?

Faith had always thought her team was committed to staying up to date and providing good care. This was the unofficial expectation that the team as a whole had of every member. They also had a culture in which they recognized themselves as visitors in patients' homes, and were courteous and respectful of the house rules of the homes they visited. They made a conscious effort to try to fit their input around patients' other activities, lifestyle and commitments. However, they were busy and frequently unable to spend as long as they would like with patients. Different people often carried out different aspects of care for each person, for example an HCA would visit one day for one task and an RN the next day for another. Thus, the team's unstated culture was that their work primarily concerned carrying out care tasks, which would be performed effectively, caringly, politely and respectfully. Faith had no argument with any aspect of that, but she was beginning to think that the person they respected could become lost in the process.

How did Faith's values affect her work? How were these values influenced by her colleagues' values?

This incident with Mr Edwards had made Faith consider what mattered to her in her work and what her values were. She thought what mattered most to her was giving good quality care, treating the people she worked with respectfully and trying to understand their perspectives. Faith believed that her work values were the importance of respect for people, colleagues and patients, and treating others as she would want to be treated herself. She also wanted people to feel that she had time for them. She liked talking to patients, hearing about their lives and getting to know the people behind the care she gave. Thus, when she looked at what she valued, it was giving good care, but also knowing and respecting the people she worked for and with. She realized that while she generally felt her work was congruent with her values, the piece that was sometimes missing was being able to have time for individuals, to get to know them as people with a past as well as a present.

Faith believed that the majority of the team she worked with shared her values about good quality care, treating people respectfully and treating others as they would want to be treated themselves. However, she was not sure that everyone valued getting to know the individual in the way she did. This was perhaps why the overall culture of care was focused on how tasks could best be completed, rather than on how people could best be understood and known. At the same time, she reflected that many of the team commented from time to time that they would like more continuity in whom they visited, so perhaps they did feel this way but, like her, had not articulated it. She realized they never discussed such matters as a team, and the overall value attributed to getting tasks completed meant that maybe they did not give themselves the opportunity to share thoughts about what was important to them.

How did the history, culture, structure, functions and power equations in Faith's team influence care provision?

Faith thought about what it was that aided but also prevented her from working in the way she would ideally like to. The most obvious thing was time. Her team had, it seemed, always been busy, hardworking and striving to provide good care. However, over time, their structure and functions had changed and the RNs had taken on particular roles while the HCAs had taken on others. This had fragmented their visits somewhat, and care had become more focused on what tasks needed doing for patients than who would visit them and how well they would get to know them.

There were no obvious power issues within the team. Although there was a team leader and a deputy, everyone seemed to feel able to suggest innovations and challenge other people's ideas. Nevertheless, below the surface, Faith thought that there were two people whose views dominated, and they were not the people who were most concerned about getting to know patients as people or respecting them. They tended to be keen to help patients to accept their perspectives, rather than finding out what patients felt about things, and were always eager to demonstrate how efficiently they managed their workloads. She thought that their views on the value of efficiency and the need to enable patients to comply with what they saw as right sometimes influenced others, especially newer staff members. They were seen as the most efficient and able and, in some respects, held the greatest unofficial power within the team, despite not being the team leader or deputy. Their values did not most closely match Faith's values.

Faith thought that while the team got on well, they spent relatively little time together and thus had limited opportunities to explore what mattered to them, as individuals and as a team.

What different types of knowledge did Faith use in practice? How did they fit into Habermas's categories of technical, practical and emancipatory knowledge?

Faith considered what informed her practice. A great deal of this was technical knowledge: she knew how the various treatments and interventions used worked and why this was the case. However, she also believed that she knew how to interact with people, diffuse difficult situations, put people at ease and encourage them to talk to her. She felt that she used this skill to gain a great deal of practical knowledge about how others saw their world, what things meant for them, what their priorities were, and how this affected what they were prepared to engage with in terms of treatment and care. Finally, in terms of emancipatory knowledge, Faith considered how far the way she worked was influenced by her own views, priorities, values and the social conditions around her. Her past work, beliefs and values meant that she was generally of the opinion that people should be listened to and respected. She felt a certain degree of frustration that she could not always achieve this in her work and perceived herself to be unable to change this, as it was linked to her team's workload. However, she also thought that the feeling she could not work as she wanted to, for reasons outside her control, meant that she sometimes distanced herself from patients. Knowing that she could not engage to the degree she wanted to, and not wanting to let her team down by having to ask for assistance with her caseload, she subconsciously failed to engage fully with the patients she visited.

An interaction Faith recently had with a patient and what influenced that interaction

Faith's caseload recently included visiting Mrs Adams, who needed to have her dressing changed, but was known to the team from previous care episodes. She generally seemed unwilling to do what she needed to do to maintain her health, and often held up the nurses' work by not being ready when they arrived. She frequently found fault with the care she received, and often announced problems as the nurses were preparing to leave, which delayed their departure. Faith knew that Mrs Adams had lived on her own since her husband died five years previously and had one son who lived in France. Faith thought that Mrs Adams was probably lonely, as she seemed to have few friends or visitors, but also that Mrs Adams did very little to help herself, because she made people feel unwelcome and rarely showed any gratitude for what they did.

When Faith arrived at the house, Mrs Adams was not ready for her. This initially irritated Faith, because she had a particularly busy schedule that day. However, she made a conscious effort not to let her workload or existing views affect her. Instead, she decided to try to understand Mrs Adams. She noticed some photograph albums on her shelf and instead of waiting impatiently, asked if she could take a look while she waited. Mrs Adams agreed, and while Faith did her dressing she asked Mrs Adams about some of the people she had seen in the photos. One was Mrs Adams' daughter, who had died at the age of 23. Faith said that she had not realized Mrs Adams had had a daughter and asked if she minded talking about her. Mrs Adams shared some tales of her daughter's life with Faith, got out several more photographs and showed her these. Faith listened and asked if Mrs Adams would be willing to show her some more photos when she came back in four days' time. When Faith got into her car, she realized that Mrs Adams had not found a difficulty to discuss when she tried to leave and her visit had lasted less time than usual. The negative influences on her interaction with Mrs Adams were that she had expected to be kept waiting, and when her expectations were met, had been irritated because of her need to get to other patients. However, she had decided to use her knowledge of herself, and how her existing beliefs about Mrs Adams and the social pressure on her to complete the visit within time influenced her, to deliberately change her mindset and course of action. This enabled her to engage in an interaction led by her wanting to know about Mrs Adams, rather than wanting to get her dressing done and leave. This seemed to result in a better quality interaction for both parties, and also made the visit quicker and more efficient than usual.

Additional resources

Practice development
www.health.nsw.gov.au/nursing/projects/Pages/practice-dev.aspx
Provides information and resources related to practice development.

www.canterbury.ac.uk/health/EnglandCentreforPracticeDevelopment/
Whatispracticedevelopment/Whatispracticedevelopment.aspx
Defines what practice development is and details some of the methodologies and methods it uses.

Person-centred care
www.rcn.org.uk/development/practice/cpd_online_learning/dignity_in_health_
care/person-centred_care
Discusses what person-centred care is and how it might be enacted.

www.science.ulster.ac.uk/inhr/public/pdf/HSE_IrelandPCPProgrammeFINAL.pdf
A report on the implementation of a model of person-centred practice.

www.effectivepractitioner.nes.scot.nhs.uk/learning-and-development/clinical-
practice/enhancing-person-centred-care.aspx
Provides a definition of person-centred care and suggests learning activities to help practitioners to develop more person-centred care.

Critical realism
http://istheory.byu.edu/wiki/Critical_realism_theory
Provides an overview of the theory of critical realism.

www.ribm.mmu.ac.uk/wps/papers/11-03.pdf
This working paper provides an evaluation of critical realist theory.

www.imi.ox.ac.uk/pdfs/wp/wp-11-42-the-positive-and-the-negative-assessing-critical-realism-and-social-constructionism-as-post-positivist-approaches-to-empirical-research-in-the-social-sciences
A working paper discussion related to critical realism.

www.maneyonline.com/loi/rea
The Journal of Critical Realism can be found here.

Critical social theory
www.redorbit.com/news/science/386919/reexamining_health_disparities_critical_social_theory_in_pediatric_nursing/
An article that applies critical social theory to nursing practice.

www127.pair.com/critical/d-ct.htm
Suggests some applications of critical theory.

www.uta.edu/huma/illuminations/kell10.htm
This article outlines the history and main tenets of critical theory.

www.uta.edu/huma/illuminations/kell5.htm
Provides a discussion of critical theory's underpinnings, history and current state.

3 Person-centred Care

Chapter overview

- The concept of personhood encompasses the physical, social, emotional, psychological and spiritual aspects of being human. However, it is the unique combination of, and interaction between, these elements that creates the whole person.
- Personhood includes the individual's ability to reflect on the past alongside considering what is happening now, and to use this to develop principles and make decisions about the future.
- Person-centredness sees the individual as a part of the wider society, with the rights and responsibilities that citizenship entails.
- While person-centred care places the person who is a patient at the centre of care, it also acknowledges the personhood of staff.
- Person-centred care can enhance patients' care experience, and job satisfaction for staff. However, achieving it requires individual and corporate effort and commitment.

Tom has worked in a post-trauma rehabilitation day service for the past year. He finds it rewarding to work with people on achieving as high a level of recovery as they can, and enjoys being part of a team where the different disciplines involved seem genuinely committed to working together to provide high-quality care. However, he is finding it increasingly frustrating when the people who use the service do not seem to want to do the things they need to do in order to maximize their recovery. He has recently been working with Jamal, a young man who was injured in a road accident and who needs ongoing rehabilitation to help him regain his mobility. Jamal's motivation to participate in rehabilitation seems limited, and Tom knows that he could make much more progress than he is making now. He understands that Jamal has undergone significant loss and has a long journey to recovery, but feels disappointed that he does not make much effort to follow the rehabilitation plans that would help him. Tom has spent a lot of time explaining to Jamal that if he does his exercises more often it will make his progress quicker.

Although Jamal agrees and appears to see this as desirable, he does not really seem interested in the day-to-day reality of doing so. Tom tries to encourage Jamal to view his therapy and goals in bite-sized chunks, so that he will not become overwhelmed and can see progress week to week. Jamal always says that he finds this helpful and promises to do his best, but then does very little.

Tom has been reading about person-centred care and practice development methodology, and wonders if these could provide answers to some of his difficulties with people like Jamal. He thinks a great deal about how each person's treatment plans can be adapted to their likely recovery trajectory and social circumstances, and spends considerable time discussing with individuals how they can best fit various aspects of therapy into their lives. Tom is committed to, and genuinely cares about, the quality of his work and those with whom he works. However, as he read about person-centredness, he began to think that he might perhaps have missed a key point.

Activity 3.1

Think about what being person centred means to you.

What it means to be a person

In order to determine whether or not he was working in a person-centred way, Tom decided that he first needed to clarify what being a person meant. He had assumed that by thinking beyond a person's physical needs to include their social, emotional, psychological and spiritual needs, he was meeting the needs of the whole person. However, as he read, he realized that this might not be enough.

There is not complete agreement on what being a person means (MacLeod and McPherson 2007, McCormack et al. 2012). Personhood can be interpreted as relating simply to membership of a biological species – being a human as distinct from the rest of the animal kingdom. However, in relation to person-centred care, it generally means more than this. The concept of personhood in this context aims to capture the range of unique human attributes, but also recognizes that seeing each of these in isolation can mean that the wholeness and complexity of personhood is lost (McCormack 2004, MacLeod and McPherson 2007). Personhood focuses on the way in which each element of a person combines with the others, making that individual a unique being, with emotions, feelings, a personality and character, as well as discrete attributes (Macleod and McPherson 2007). Each person is also influenced by their family, cultural background, life experiences, the roles they take on, their relationships with themselves and others, their spirituality, secret life and perceived future (Macleod and McPherson 2007). A person is therefore much more than the sum of their parts.

Practice pointer 3.1

Each person's unique self is influenced by their physical characteristics, social situation, emotional disposition, spirituality, psychological status, life experiences, family members and situation, culture, history, relationships with self and others and perceived future. The unique combination of these in each individual makes up the person.

It had always been Tom's belief that he should provide care that considered the social, psychological, spiritual and emotional, as well as physical, elements of a person's injury and rehabilitation. He now began to wonder, though, if he had looked at discrete parts of the person, and missed how these combined to make each individual respond in a unique way to their circumstances. With Jamal, he had assumed that a young man who had been employed in a good job and studying part time at university would be keen to maximize his rehabilitation. However, he had never really considered what other factors in Jamal's life, personality and character might influence this. This included whether the life and focus that he was aiming to enable Jamal to regain was what he had wanted in the past, or wanted now, and whether Jamal's usual approach to life was fairly laissez faire and mirrored in his approach to rehabilitation. He had also not really taken into account the spiritual aspects of Jamal's personhood. While he had always been respectful of Jamal's religious beliefs and practices, Tom had not considered how Jamal's private spiritual thoughts might affect his perceptions of his injury and rehabilitation, or how these might be affecting his spiritual self and his perceptions of the meaning and purpose of his life (Rieg et al. 2006, Barnum 2010). Tom realized that he knew very little about who Jamal was, as a person, and how this might affect his rehabilitation. This might be creating frustration on his part, as the Jamal he assumed he was working with might not be the person he was actually encountering.

McCormack (2004) suggests that personhood includes the ability to reflect on the past and what is happening now, in order to make decisions about one's preferences, purposes and principles, and guide current and future decision making. This freedom of thought is distinct from the individual's physical abilities, and exists even when their ability to act on their views, preferences or desires is limited. McCormack (2004) describes this aspect of personhood as a 'moral personality' that gives every person, regardless of their physical needs or abilities, an intrinsic worth and requires them to be treated with dignity and respect. Person-centred care places this unique person, with all their complexities and free will to think, decide and choose, at the centre of care.

Tom thought about whether his frustrations with people who did not seem motivated to follow their rehabilitation programmes arose from him not appreciating that this might be a choice they had made, based on their preferences, desires and principles. This also made him consider whether he saw the people he worked with as a part of their wider social context, and as citizens outside their rehabilitation encounters.

Activity 3.2

Think about someone you cared for the last time you were at work. What do you know about them as a person?

Practice pointer 3.2

Personhood recognizes people's ability to:

- develop principles, purposes and preferences based on what has gone before and what is happening now
- use these preferences, purposes and principles to guide the decisions they make
- have freedom of thought and choice, even when their ability to act on their thoughts and choices is limited.

Personhood and citizenship

While person-centredness recognizes the uniqueness of individuals and how their immediate social situation contributes to who they are, people are also a part of a wider society, which influences who they are and what is available to them. This links with the concept of citizenship, where each person is viewed not just as themselves, or a member of their circle of family, friends and colleagues, but as a part of a larger collective group (Bartlett and O'Connor 2007, Perron et al. 2010). Being a citizen means that the individual has equality and rights, but also responsibilities and duties (Bartlett and O'Connor 2007, Perron et al. 2010). It goes beyond seeing the individual, to seeing the corporate, and the effects of power on individuals, groups and society as a whole (Bartlett and O'Connor 2007). This incorporation of citizenship into debates on person-centredness echoes practice development methodology's underpinnings of critical social theory and critical realism, as discussed in Chapter 2. Here, the context in which events occur, but also the power individuals and groups hold in particular situations are seen as important in understanding what happens and why it happens (Freeman and Vasconcelos 2010, Bevan et al. 2012, Lapum et al. 2012).

Considering personhood or citizenship alone is not enough for person-centred practice. Citizenship tends to see citizens as equal, and in so doing can imply that people are all the same – having, and therefore wanting, the same rights, responsibilities, duties and power (Bartlett and O'Connor 2007). Personhood, on the other hand, while focusing on individuality does not explore power relations, responsibilities and duties. Thus, neither concept fully grasps the complexities of being a person who is a part of a wider society (Bartlett and O'Connor 2007, Perron et al. 2010). As a result, personhood and citizenship both need to be considered in person-centred practice.

Practice pointer 3.3

Citizenship includes considering individual and corporate equality, rights, responsibilities, duties and power.

Tom could see how both citizenship and personhood were key elements of what made up the people with whom he worked. He also thought that perhaps he did not always fully consider their citizenship and personhood in his encounters with them. He had always tried to approach his relationship with Jamal on an equal footing, was careful not to appear coercive, and to be respectful of the choices that Jamal made, even when he found them frustrating. Nonetheless, he had not really considered how Jamal's level of empowerment, both in society and in healthcare, affected his rehabilitation. This included Jamal's previous responsibilities, rights and power, his perception of these, and how these were affected by his current impairments. It could also involve how Jamal perceived Tom's power, as the professional, and how this might influence their interactions. Tom had always thought that as Jamal was not generally compliant with his rehabilitation plans, he did not feel intimidated or disempowered in their relationship. He now reflected that feelings of disempowerment might mean that Jamal did not feel able to express his thoughts or feelings about his rehabilitation, especially if they differed from Tom's. His apparent agreement might, therefore, simply represent a perceived need to behave deferentially towards a professional, rather than meaning that Jamal really agreed with Tom, intended, or felt able, to follow his instructions.

It also struck Tom that he had not really explored Jamal's responsibilities and rights in the choices he made. He had effectively set himself up as the expert, whose views should be followed, and in so doing seemed to have taken on responsibility for whether or not Jamal complied with his recommendations. He had not discussed with Jamal his right, but also responsibility, to make and live with his decisions regarding his rehabilitation.

Tom now thought that he had probably not been as person centred in his dealings with Jamal as he had always assumed he was. This led him to consider exactly what person-centredness in care meant.

Activity 3.3

How might patients perceive you in your work role? How might this affect what they tell you and how they respond to care?

Practice pointer 3.4

Person-centredness includes personhood and citizenship; looking at the person as a unique individual, but also how they function as a part of society as a whole, with rights as well as responsibilities.

What is person-centredness in care?

Person-centredness in care acknowledges each person's uniqueness and centres care on that person as an individual and a citizen (Manley et al. 2011, Parish 2012). While meeting a person's physical needs will always be a vital part of healthcare provision, person-centred care focuses on what makes a person who they are, and how care can be provided so as to best achieve what matters to them in relation to their health. Tom now appreciated that seeing the interplay between a person's physical health and other aspects of their life and wellbeing was good, but was not the same as person-centredness. It concerned identifying how their physical health needs could best be met and matching this, as far as possible, to various other elements of their life. However, the meeting of the person's physical needs, as defined by the professionals providing care, was the focus.

Central to person-centred care is getting to know the person so that they, with all their unique characteristics including their hopes, dreams, goals, values and personality, and the combination of these that makes them who they are, are at the centre of care (McCance et al. 2008, Cloninger 2011, Thornton 2011). This person's rights, but also responsibilities, are at the core of decision-making processes, with care radiating from them and linking to every part of them, at every point, rather than circling around them. Tom felt that this was exactly what he had missed. He thought back to a recent discussion he had had with Jamal about what made it difficult for him to do his exercises. Jamal had laughed and said: 'I just never seem to get around to it!' Tom had asked if Jamal found his lack of quick progress demotivating, and whether it was difficult for him to find a reason to do his exercises. Jamal had replied that he could not really say what the problem was: he always intended to do his exercises later in the day, but found that later never happened. Tom also recalled overhearing Jamal laughing and saying to another person: 'I always used to do my university assignments at the last minute!' Tom realized that perhaps what he had missed was that Jamal would always delay doing things, because this was a personal trait, a part of the complex mix of what made him Jamal, and nothing to do with his injury or motivation for rehabilitation. He had never asked Jamal: 'Are you like this with other things too?' or 'How do you usually persuade yourself to do things you know you need and really want to do, but put off?'

Person-centredness is not just about understanding what a person is experiencing at present, but also getting to know what they have been, experienced and valued in the past and hope for in the future (McKeown et al. 2010, Thornton 2011). Tom had taken a great deal of time to think about every aspect of the Jamal he saw in front of him – his health, social situation, studies, employment, what seemed to have been his interests and goals at the time of his accident, and how his accident would have affected these. However, he had never asked a great deal about anything beyond the first two or three weeks before Jamal's accident. He did not know Jamal's history in terms of how he had become who he was, what he had experienced and valued in the past, and what this meant for who he was and who he wanted to be. He had not considered how this would influence the choices Jamal made and how he expressed them – what he said, what he did not say and his behaviours. Tom had been encouraging Jamal to work on his rehabilitation programme so that he could return to work and university, but did not know why Jamal had chosen his job or university course, and whether these were ever a key part of his life. He had not really thought about whether Jamal's past experience would make him someone who wanted to work hard to maximize his recovery, or be a passive recipient of whatever happened. He did not know if Jamal usually expected success, failure, or a middle point, and what influenced his expectations. He was also not aware of whether Jamal was generally proactive in taking responsibility for his own situation, or whether he allowed others to dictate this. Tom now thought that by considering Jamal's personhood and citizenship in more depth, Jamal's rehabilitation, and his own job satisfaction, might be improved. However, he felt that he also needed to clarify what this would mean he should do, in practice.

Practice pointer 3.5

Person-centredness focuses on the person:

* with unique characteristics, hopes, dreams, goals, values, strengths, weaknesses and a personality
* physically, mentally, emotionally, socially and spiritually
* as a part of society with rights and responsibilities
* with a past, and expectations for the future.

Person-centred care

Person-centred care focuses on getting to know the person who is a patient, including their history, values, beliefs, priorities, preferences, current situation, future aspirations and how they make sense of what is happening to them (McCormack and McCance 2006, Manley et al. 2011, van den Pol-Grevelink et al. 2012). It also encompasses considering how the person's own, and other people's, perceptions of their place in society, power, rights and responsibilities affects who they are or see themselves as being. It requires practitioners to effectively enter another person's world and see how they see things (van den Pol-Grevelink et al. 2012). It does not require them to agree with these perceptions or adopt them, but to be able to view matters through the eyes of the person they are working with, and appreciate how this shapes their reality and choices.

Tom considered this, and concluded that he had not really been person centred in his encounters with Jamal. He had focused on what he knew Jamal could achieve, or thought he would be happiest achieving. He realized that his disappointments in his work with Jamal might largely be caused by him not thinking about the person who Jamal was beyond the person who presented at rehabilitation. He also reflected that while he had always apparently respected Jamal's right to decline to participate fully in his rehabilitation, he had not really accepted this view or considered what the reasons for it might be. Tom's frustration was that he was expecting Jamal to achieve his goals, not Jamal's, and was effectively also taking responsibility for Jamal achieving these.

McCance et al. (2008) and McCarthy (2006) identify that person-centredness goes beyond treating people well and speaking to them respectfully, to exploring and respecting their perceptions, needs and decisions. This was something Tom felt he could work on to reduce the difficulties he encountered with people like Jamal, provide them with a better experience of rehabilitation, but also facilitate them making choices that would be beneficial to them, as individuals. Tom had always, even when exasperated by Jamal, been courteous. However, he had accepted what he now thought were probably fairly superficial explanations for why Jamal was not doing his rehabilitation work, because he had never engaged with him in a way that encouraged any other level of discussion. The dialogue had always been around why Jamal did not do his exercises and what the effect of this would be, not what he wanted to be, do and achieve, how this was affected by his injuries, and how the suggested therapies might contribute to him developing that Jamal.

It occurred to Tom that he had always put his own view forward to Jamal as the professional, or expert, view but had probably not explored, with Jamal or himself, why he personally did or did not recommend things. His training and existing beliefs were such that he had always presented these professional views as a third party, without any input about himself. As well as not learning about the person who was Jamal, he realized that he had not engaged with Jamal as a person, only as a professional.

Practice pointer 3.6

Person-centred care does not require people to agree with each other: it requires practitioners to try to understand patients' perspectives, what matters to them, and how their views have been formed.

Respecting the individual as a person requires professionals to accept their right to self-determination, even when the choices they make differ from what professionals see as the best course of action (McCance et al. 2008, McGilton et al. 2012). This does not mean, however, that professionals should withdraw from decision-making situations. Rather, they should be prepared to engage in sharing their experience, knowledge, evidence, views and interpretations in order to assist people to understand their options and the likely consequences of the choices they make (Manley et al. 2011). Professionals should not present their own opinions, values or beliefs in a coercive manner (GMC 2012). However, McCormack (2003) identifies that a professional explaining their own values and perspectives to patients need not be coercive. Instead, it can be a means of acknowledging the person-hood of both parties, and also encourage patients to discuss how their perspectives shape the choices they wish to make. It may help each person to understand the other's viewpoint and offer additional, potentially helpful insights to both parties. Thus, person-centred care gives practitioners a key role in sharing with patients in the decision-making process (McCormack et al. 2010, Manley et al. 2011, McKay et al. 2012, van den Pol-Grevelink et al. 2012). This shared decision making, in which patients and profession-als engage in genuine and open sharing of information, perspectives and understanding of treatment, care and management options, is a key aspect of person-centred care (Wiley et al. 2014).

Person-centred care requires practitioners not just to understand and respect, but also act on what the individual patient values (McCormack and McCance 2006, McKay et al. 2012, van den Pol-Grevelink et al. 2012). This includes supporting the person to assert their choices, regardless of whether the professional agrees with these, and without an obligation for them to agree with them (Manley et al. 2011). Nonetheless, it has the potential to create a dilemma if patients want to take a path that requires actions professionals are not willing, or able, to engage in. The recognition and respect for each individual's personhood and citizenship seen in person-centred care is particularly important in this situation. By sharing their perspectives, it should be possible for practitioners to be open, honest and clear about what, as a professional, a person and a citizen, they can and cannot be involved in. For example, the professional's responsibility and duty as a citizen of a particular country, as well as their professional responsibility and duty, means that certain activities are not permissible for them, regardless of the desires of another individual.

Tom could see some good reasons to alter the way he approached his work. However, he still wondered if this really would make things better for all concerned. He felt instinctively that it should, but wanted to consider this in more depth.

Practice pointer 3.7

• Person-centredness recognizes the personhood and citizenship of practitioners as well as patients.
• To achieve person-centred care, practitioners need to acknowledge their own personhood and citizenship.

Activity 3.4

Think about an instance where you and a patient had different views about their treatment or care. How did you resolve this?

Why person-centred care is beneficial

The idea of adopting a more person-centred approach to practice somewhat challenged Tom's pride in the high quality of his knowledge and technical skills, which felt slightly threatening. However, as he explored person-centredness, he realized that the focus on knowing people did not detract from the importance of sound knowledge, technical skills and competence (MacLeod and McPherson 2007). Rather, it meant that he could channel these so that they were focused on the individual with whom he was working (McGilton et al. 2012). The higher his level of knowledge and skills, the more confident he would be in discussing different perspectives, options and possible outcomes from different approaches, and working with people to tailor provision to their unique situations. In Tom's work with Jamal, for instance, it would not be acceptable for him to have less knowledge or skills. These were all still essential. What was needed was for them to be made available alongside knowledge of Jamal as a person, which would enable them to jointly plan the best way for Tom's technical skills and knowledge to be used to help Jamal to achieve what mattered to him. It would mean that Tom's expertise was more effectively used, in helping Jamal and others to achieve what was important to them. At the moment, Tom's skills and knowledge were being used to plan how Jamal's needs, as identified by Tom, could be met, but this might not lead to an outcome that Jamal wanted or valued.

Person-centredness would not necessarily lead to the achievement of the outcomes that Tom had previously valued most highly, such as ensuring that individuals regained maximum functional ability in a good time frame, or were able to return to work. It would, however, lead to outcomes that he did, now that he had considered it, value but had not formally recognized before. These ranged from enhanced care provision in small day-to-day issues, to enabling people to achieve outcomes that mattered to them. The small parts of this might include having conversations that were meaningful for the person (Edvardsson et al. 2010). Tom usually chatted to Jamal about things that he seemed interested in, but learning more about who Jamal was might make these casual conversations easier and the time they spent together more congenial. At another level, if Jamal felt that Tom was genuinely interested in him, it could make conversations about his goals, concerns and motivations easier for him to enter into.

As well as meaning that care is focused on outcomes that matter to patients, which is likely to enhance their satisfaction with care, working in a person-centred way has, in some cases, been shown to have a positive effect on practitioners' job satisfaction (van den Pol-Grevelink et al. 2012). Tom could see how working in a more person-centred way might be less frustrating for him. Being able to work with individuals to achieve what they felt was best for them, not what seemed best to him, and enabling them to own and take responsibility for these decisions would probably make his work more satisfying and less stressful. Tom also enjoyed a challenge, and liked making innovations in his work. Working in a person-centred way offered him the opportunity for every encounter to be the start of a challenge, in which he and the person concerned explored approaches that were uniquely designed for that individual. This also meant that Tom would work with each person on an innovative, personalized piece of practice.

Tom did not feel that his core beliefs and values had altered completely. His existing desire to provide high-quality care had been adjusted to focus on the person who was accessing rehabilitation, rather than on how that person could be enabled to accommodate their prescribed therapy. He had also shifted his thinking from being responsible for the person's recovery to being responsible for allowing them to make informed choices about their recovery. Tom was now convinced that person-centredness was what was missing from his work, but was aware he would need to cultivate new habits of thinking and working to enable him to achieve this day to day. This would require some effort on his part and he would need support in it.

Practice pointer 3.8

Person-centred care:

- does not detract from the importance of technical skills and knowledge
- enables practitioners to combine their knowledge of the person and their technical skills and knowledge to provide care that centres on the individual and the outcomes they value
- can enhance staff satisfaction as well as patients' experiences.

Activity 3.5

What would the benefits of being person centred in your practice be? Would there be any disadvantages?

What is needed to achieve person-centredness?

McCormack et al. (2010), Manley et al. (2011) and McGilton et al. (2012) identify that consistently providing person-centred care requires individuals and workplaces to have a philosophy and culture that subscribes to and really values this ethos. Tom thought that if he was the only person on the unit trying to work in a more person-centred way, his good intentions would soon be eroded and he would, inadvertently, revert to his previous way of thinking and acting. This led him to consider what would need to exist in his workplace in order for him to succeed in working in a person-centred way.

A key part of achieving person-centred care is knowing people. It is impossible to know people without having the skills to gather information about them and develop the level of trust that will enable them to be honest about what matters to them, and how far interventions or care are helping them (MacLeod and McPherson 2007, McCormack et al. 2010). In order for this to happen, as well as developing their communication and observation skills, practitioners need the time and ability to reflect on information they have gathered, consider and discuss what matters to the individual, and how this can be translated into treatment and care (Manley et al. 2011). Tom felt that his workplace already saw it as important to spend time with patients and work thoroughly with them on their rehabilitation plans. However, the approach taken to conversations, and the way in which people reflected on and used the information gained, might need to alter.

High-quality care was certainly valued on the unit, and time and funding for ongoing professional development were seen as an important investment. Nonetheless, as Chapter 4 will discuss, to develop more person-centred care, this would need to include the time and resources to enable people to develop cognitive, emotional and reflective skills, as well as technical skills and knowledge (McGilton et al. 2012).

Practising in a person-centred way can require a degree of risk taking. Getting to know and understand patients can seem risky in terms of involvement, fear of loss of objectivity, and risk to one's own emotional wellbeing (MacLeod and McPherson 2007). Real person-centredness also requires trust and openness to exist between individuals, and professionals may fear their own emotions, beliefs, values and humanity being uncovered in discussions of this nature (MacLeod and McPherson 2007). In order to offer person-centred care, practitioners have to feel enabled, and permitted, to give of themselves as people and to take risks (Manley et al. 2009, Finset 2011). Tom believed that while he and his colleagues were generally treated, and treated one another as well as patients, respectfully and considerately, they were not really encouraged to engage as people in their interactions with patients. This would be an aspect of the unit's culture that would need to be developed in order for person-centred care to be consistently provided.

Tom had never considered his workplace to be coercive or disempowering. However, he now acknowledged that the unstated goal was to enable patients to comply with practitioners' recommendations, not to explore with patients their personal goals and how practitioners could help them to achieve those. This was something else that he thought the unit would need to work on in order for person-centred practice to become a day-to-day reality there.

Tom was uncertain whether his colleagues would want to move towards working in a more person-centred way. He thought that it was likely that some people would, but he would need to plan how best to approach discussing this, so as not to detract from the many positive aspects of the unit that neither he nor anyone else would want to lose.

Practice pointer 3.9

• Being person centred requires time, effort, a recognition of one's own humanity, the ability to take risks, and the desire to develop a person-centred approach.
• For person-centred care to succeed, this has to be the dominant ethos in a workplace's philosophy and culture.

Activity 3.6

What in your workplace would enhance or inhibit person-centred care?

Summary

Tom had now identified that he wanted to alter the way he worked, so that the people whose rehabilitation he facilitated and their views, priorities, values, ambitions, hopes and beliefs were central to the care he provided. This included encounters being focused on seeking to understand people and what mattered to them, based on their past, their present and their anticipated future. It also meant seeing people as citizens, with rights, but also responsibilities, for making choices. As well as seeing patients as people, Tom now saw the value of acknowledging his own personhood in his practice. However, he also recognized that in order for this to become a reality, some aspects of the current ethos of his workplace would need to alter. This was likely to include developing a culture of learning and development that was slightly different from that which currently existed.

Case scenario

For the past seven months Alex has been working at a unit that provides daycare for people who have moderate learning disabilities. He is not really enjoying working there. He does not think that the people who use the unit are mistreated, but feels that they are not really viewed as individuals, with all that this entails. The philosophy the unit subscribes to is described as 'client-centred care', but Alex is questioning whether this is what happens in reality. These thoughts have led him to review what he considers being client, or person, centred to mean.

What being person centred means to Alex

Alex sees being person centred as meaning that he focuses what he does on who the person he is dealing with is. This includes their:

• preferences, such how they like their tea or coffee, the way they prefer to dress, the activities they enjoy

- physical and cognitive capabilities
- emotional responses
- ways of expressing themselves
- way of processing information
- values and spiritual beliefs.

It also includes what has happened to them in the past and what they want to do in the future. This might include weekend activities, holidays and other ambitions. Seeing the person means, to Alex, looking at how these things all add up together to make the person as a whole, and trying to tailor the care he provides to that person. Thinking about what person-centredness means has caused Alex to consider what he actually knows about the people who use the day centre.

Alex thought about someone he worked with regularly and what he knew about them as a person

Alex regularly works with Billy. He knows that Billy is 25 years old and lives with his mother and father. He has two older siblings who are both married and live away from the area, but visit their parents and Billy quite regularly. Billy occasionally visits them, but it is difficult for them to accommodate him. He has five nieces and nephews, whom he talks about enthusiastically. He has a good memory and can recall what he does with his nephews and nieces in great detail. Billy likes anything to do with sport, but especially football and cricket. He dislikes animals, because he finds them unpredictable. Billy thinks about things a great deal, but is quite slow at processing information. He finds walking difficult, and has some hearing impairment, but enjoys any opportunity to help out. He values being able to be helpful and sees his desire to help others as one of his good qualities. This can be difficult for staff because Billy helping does not always make things easier to complete. If Billy is discouraged from helping, it upsets him, sometimes apparently out of proportion to the task he had been denied participation in.

There are many parts of who Billy is that Alex thinks might contribute to him being upset by not being able to help. His hearing loss and way of processing information probably make it difficult for him to understand why he has been asked not to help. He also finds speaking difficult, especially if he feels upset, so it is hard for him to express himself. This could make him feel frustrated and angry as he cannot fully understand or be understood, which, along with the disappointment he feels at not being able to do something he enjoys, values and sees as a core part of who he is, all contribute to his distress. Billy likes being with people, so helping out also gives him company and a sense of worth. Being refused the opportunity to help could feel like a rejection of what he sees himself as standing for.

This is just one part of what Alex knows of Billy. He also suspects that how Billy perceives the staff on the unit may contribute to his responses in certain situations.

How might the people Alex works with perceive him in his work role? How might this affect what they tell him and how they respond to care?

Alex thought about Billy and his parents, and how they might view the staff at the day unit. Billy's parents generally seemed grateful for the care the unit provided, but did not always appear completely satisfied with how things went for Billy. On days when Billy was upset, they looked unhappy, but never questioned staff. Alex assumed that they too had to deal with Billy's disappointments and knew how difficult this could be. However, he also wondered if they perceived staff as being busy and perhaps not really having the time to consider Billy as an individual, so that any discussion of what had happened would not be worthwhile. They might also view staff as being in a position of power, and not want to be seen to be complaining, in case what care Billy had was reduced. Equally, they might feel that the unit was part of a large impersonal system that could not be changed and that challenging, questioning or even suggesting amendments to how Billy's needs were managed would therefore be futile. On one occasion, Alex had asked Billy's mother if she had any hints she could share with him on the best way to work with Billy when he was upset. He had genuinely wanted to know, but it had taken a while for her to see this, and she initially deferred to his expertise in how to handle 'people like Billy'. When he eventually convinced her to share her ideas, they included some useful insights.

Alex thought about an instance where he and Billy's mother had different views about Billy's time at the daycare unit and how they resolved this

On one occasion, Billy had been due to attend the unit on a day when a trip to the local farm was planned. Billy's mother had indicated that Billy should go as it would be useful for him to become a little less extreme in his responses to animals. Alex had wondered if this would be useful, as Billy always seemed to be terrified by animals and became distressed by any contact with them. He had said that perhaps on this occasion Billy should not participate in the visit. They had discussed why Billy's mother considered it important for Billy to get used to animals, and she had explained that his nephews and nieces always wanted to show him their pets, and that it would be useful if he could become less averse to them. She had felt that a trip to the farm, where experienced people would be available to help him, might be a good way to do this. Although Alex disagreed, Billy's mother had been uncharacteristically determined and eventually it had been agreed that Billy would go. Billy had not enjoyed the trip, and the staff member with him had had a difficult day.

Thinking back, Alex realized that the discussion had only really focused on Billy's aversion to animals, not on Billy as a person, his mother as a person, Alex as a person, and the many things that made up their views, preferences and priorities. He reflected that he had not considered what Billy's mother did when Billy was at the unit, and how his time there was slotted in with her other needs, commitments and priorities, and those of her family. He had also not shared his concerns outside Billy's needs; for example, that he felt it would be difficult to manage Billy's emotions while also caring for other people on the trip, and he was not confident that he knew the best way to manage Billy in this situation. Other negotiated options might have existed if both parties had been able to be more open about the breadth of factors underpinning their views.

Alex considered the benefits and disadvantages of being person centred in his practice

Being more person centred would mean that Alex and his colleagues under-stood more fully what mattered to people, and what would make their time at the unit useful and positive for them. It would be likely to mean that the people who used the day unit had a more enjoyable and profitable time there and might reduce episodes of what was seen as problem behaviour. This would, in turn, probably enhance job satisfaction for staff. Alex also felt that this way of working would be beneficial for relatives and carers. Working with Billy's family in a more person-centred way would enable him to discuss and better understand their preferences, beliefs, values, expectations, history, social situ-ation, and how Billy and the support he received affected these. If he was also prepared to share a little more of himself as a person, it would make it easier for him to explore with them the difficulties, differences of opinion and chal-lenges they all faced, because they could interact more freely.

One challenge to Alex and his workplace achieving person-centred care would be time. It took time to get to know individuals. It also took effort and involved the risk of the unknown. The unknown included how existing routines, roles and status (both formal and informal) might change if the way they approached their work altered. In addition, the awareness of oneself and others, which person-centredness requires, could be uncomfortable for those who were not used to this approach.

What in Alex's workplace would enhance or inhibit person-centred care?

A major issue in developing person-centred practice in Alex's workplace would be time, both for developing this approach to care and practising in this way every day. People might not feel confident working in this way and would need to develop their skills and confidence in it. Some people were likely to find questioning the ethos of their work challenging or threatening. The biggest issue in whether or not person-centred care was developed would, however, be whether people wanted to progress towards working in this way. The manager of the unit seemed unlikely to be enthusiastic, which could be a major barrier to other people adopting this approach.

In terms of what would help the development of person-centred provision, Alex believed that several staff members already did their best to work in this way and would like the opportunity to develop it further. One of them was a well-liked member of staff, who would probably be influential in how other people responded to any suggestion for altering the way they worked. The unit had busy times and quieter times, so they might be able to use the quieter times to develop and plan their ideas about working in a more person-centred way.

The views and expectations of the people who used the unit and their families would also be important factors in whether or not person-centred care could be achieved. Alex thought that most of the people who used the unit would enjoy a more person-centred approach, although they might initially find any consequent changes in routines or approaches unsettling. This latter point might, in turn, make staff waver in their enthusiasm for it. Although he thought that most families would appreciate a more person-centred approach, he could identify one or two who never seemed to want to interact with staff and might find this approach rather demanding. Again, this might feed into any disinclination by staff to alter the way they worked.

While the practicalities of exploring a more person-centred approach to provision would require attention, Alex felt that the human factors would be the more challenging and would most affect the achievement of person-centred care.

Additional resources

www.health.org.uk/areas-of-work/topics/person-centred-care
Discusses why person-centred care matters and how it can become a reality.

www.rcn.org.uk/development/practice/cpd_online_learning/dignity_in_health_care/person-centred_care
Discusses what person-centred care is and how it can be achieved.

www.health.vic.gov.au/older/toolkit/02PersonCentredPractice/docs/Guide%20to%20implentating%20Person%20centred%20practice.pdf
A guide on how to implement person-centred practice.

4 Creating a Culture of Learning and Development

Chapter overview

- Practice development methodology aims to develop a culture in which people engage in active learning, with their own practice as its central focus. Within this, reflective learning and high challenge/high support methods are key strategies.
- Appreciative inquiry can be a useful approach to use in developing practice because it focuses on the strengths of individuals, teams and organizations, rather than their deficits.
- Individuals and teams developing the skills of reflection and reflexivity are important elements of sustaining person-centred practice development.

Sahib is the manager of a community mental health team whose stated ethos is that they work in partnership with patients and their families. There has been some discussion within the team lately around the idea of person-centred care, and whether they achieve this. The assumption seems to be that implicit in the team's statement of partnership working is that their work is person centred. However, Sahib is not sure about this. He is fairly confident that in the vast majority of cases, his team are courteous and respectful to the people with whom they work. He also thinks that they generally work conscientiously with individuals to reach agreements on the care and support they will be provided with, and how professionals will work with them towards achieving improvements in their health. However, having read about person-centred care, he is not sure that he and his team really work in a way that acknowledges each person's uniqueness and centres care on that person as an individual and what matters to them (Manley et al. 2011, Parish 2012).

Sahib wants to explore with the team whether they feel that they could develop a more person-centred approach to their work, and has been considering the means he might employ to achieve this. Practice development methodology seems to him to be a potentially useful approach, so he has been looking at the methods it uses. He has discovered that these focus on practitioners actively participating in learning from and in practice situations (McCormack 2006). The participatory element of this appeals to Sahib because it is consistent with the approach he usually takes to managing the team. His intention is that everyone should participate in decision making, feel listened to and valued. In terms of developing practice, he likes to encourage team members to think of ideas or innovations they would like to try, rather than him dictating what should be done. That any learning that occurs should be directly related to his team's own practice also seems to Sahib to be important. He believes that while most of his team will, in principle, agree that person-centred care is the ideal, what will be essential to the development of person-centred practice will be whether they are able and willing to work in this way.

Sahib is aware that his team work hard and do a lot of things well. He likes the idea of the team developing a more person-centred way of working, but wants to approach this in a manner that will not be perceived to criticize or devalue their current commitment and achievements. He has come across the principles of appreciative inquiry, and intends to use these to explore the idea of developing a more person-centred approach to care with his team.

Activity 4.1

What does the team you work with do well?

Practice pointer 4.1

Practice development methodology uses methods that emphasize:

- participation
- learning from practice situations
- learning in practice situations.

Appreciative inquiry

While Sahib wants to challenge himself and his team, he considers it important for this to happen in a supportive, positive manner. He wants the focus to be on inspiring them to provide even better care, not to make them feel despondent about the quality of the care they currently give. He thinks that appreciative inquiry will be useful in this respect, because it involves focusing on the strengths of individuals, teams and organizations and what they can do, rather than on what has gone wrong or what cannot be done (Moore 2008, Parish 2012). Its assumption is that every organization has something that works well, is effective and successful. Sahib thinks that this approach could be useful for working with his team: he wants to celebrate what they are achieving, respectful and diligent care, but move this on to incorporate person-centredness.

Appreciative inquiry effectively approaches developing practice from the opposite perspective to problem-based thinking. In problem-based thinking, the focus is on discussing problems that have occurred. This can mean that the efforts that individuals, teams and organizations have made, and their strengths, are devalued or missed (Walsh et al. 2009). Instead of presenting his team with the problem that the care they currently provide is not as person centred as it could be, Sahib wants to express appreciation of their high-quality work and their commitment to individual patients and one another. He then aims to explore how they can use these positive characteristics and achievements to move their practice on even further. He does not intend to ignore any problems that exist, but the primary aim will be to focus on the team's considerable strengths and, by so doing, create ways to enhance care without losing what they value and do well (Moore 2008).

Appreciative inquiry focuses on allowing people to describe what they value in their current work and, from this, share their visions of what could make things even better. This process is intended to empower individuals and teams to creatively construct a better future, based on their strengths, rather than focusing on how they can remedy deficits (Moore 2008). Sahib considers this to be consistent with the principles of practice development methodology in terms of focusing on the experiences and perspectives of individual people, empowerment and critical creativity (McCormack 2006, McCormack et al. 2006, Wilson and McCormack 2006, Manley et al. 2013a). He thinks that using the principles of appreciative inquiry will enable his team to enjoy the freedom to develop a more person-centred approach to care based on their strengths and what they would like to achieve.

Practice pointer 4.2

Appreciative inquiry:

- focuses on the strengths of individuals, teams and organizations and what they do well
- assumes that every individual and organization does something that is effective and successful
- uses identified strengths to develop practice.

Appreciative inquiry, like practice development methodology, sees development as an ongoing task, which becomes a way of life for the individuals and teams concerned (McCormack et al. 2010). This is something that Sahib can see is important. His knowledge of person-centred care suggests that, to be successful, it requires a culture in which this is a way of working, rather than a task or aspect of work to be completed. He also recognizes that any change in practice, whatever its nature, needs to become embedded in the workplace culture and developed further over time, in order to be sustained (Golden 2006, Virani et al. 2009, Balasubramanian et al. 2010). He therefore considers it necessary to use methods that will enable his team to initiate, but also sustain and further develop, a person-centred approach to care. To achieve this, practice development methodology focuses on developing cultures in which the norm and expectation is ongoing, person-centred learning.

Practice pointer 4.3

Practice development methodology aims to create a culture of ongoing, practice-focused, person-centred learning.

Learning cultures

Learning cultures refer to cultures in which the dominant ethos includes a commitment to ongoing learning. However, for this learning to be focused on developing practice, it has to be based around what happens in the practice setting. For it to be consistent with developing person-centred practice, it has to be learning that is focused on developing person-centredness in the practice setting. The aim of developing a person-centred learning culture is, therefore, to develop a culture in which the dominant ethos includes ongoing, practice-focused learning directed at making care more person centred. In this type of culture, practitioners continually challenge their current practice, consider what influences this, and explore how it could become more person centred (Dewing 2010).

Learning that is based on the practice of the individual or team in question begins from where they are. A team that already works in a relatively person-centred way can still be challenged to explore areas where this could be honed even further. Equally, an area of practice that currently has very little person-centred working can begin to consider how they could start to move in this direction. Sahib thinks that this approach of taking his team from where they are at present has a natural link with the principles of appreciative inquiry. It will enable him to acknowledge that his team's work is already of a high standard, but then explore whether they can build on this to do things even better and move to a more person-centred focus.

Activity 4.2

How could your team use their strengths to develop a more person-centred approach to care?

Practice pointer 4.4

Developing a person-centred learning culture begins from where individuals and teams are. The key issue is not whether an individual or team is already working in a person-centred way, but whether they are prepared to challenge themselves and others in order to become more person centred.

A key part of developing this type of learning culture is the use of processes that enable individuals and teams to consider whether the beliefs, values, behaviours and systems they currently work with are consistent with person-centred care. These processes also need to create the opportunity for individuals and teams to think about what might be done to achieve a more person-centred focus and the part they need to play in this (McCormack et al. 2009). Sahib thinks that such processes are what he will need to use to explore with his team whether their values, priorities and practice are person centred. He suspects that almost everyone in his team would ideally like to practise in a person-centred manner, but feel constrained in some way from achieving this. These constraints may include people's beliefs, values, perceptions of themselves and others, but also perceptions of professional values, perceived requirements, the practicalities of their workload, their established way of working and their personal needs. Sahib thinks that using a structure that allows in-depth exploration of these issues will be the right way to begin the process of developing a more person-centred approach to care.

For a culture of learning to develop, the majority of Sahib's team will need to become engaged in, and committed to, learning from and in practice. He wonders if this will present him with a challenge. The team already routinely engage in supervision, debriefing and support following particular incidents. So Sahib thinks they will have some familiarity with this approach to learning from practice, although the focus will be different. Instead of considering particular actions or situations, he will be asking people to think about their whole approach to care provision, and challenging the assumptions, values, beliefs and taken-for-granted rights and wrongs of this.

While most of the staff in Sahib's team are keen to learn and try new ideas, these have, to date, generally focused on learning about new interventions and seeing how these work with individual people. The approach he is considering using to develop person-centred care is quite different; it will involve people challenging themselves to think about the fundamental principles on which they base their work. Sahib thinks that at least two people on his team may not be keen to engage in this type of learning.

Thus, although Sahib believes his team will probably be familiar with identifying and reflectively discussing particular practice situations, they may be less comfortable with in-depth exploration of the basis of the care they provide. This is one reason why he considers that using the principles of appreciative inquiry will be valuable. He hopes this will enable people to begin by exploring what in their current values, beliefs and priorities are good and can be built on to develop person-centred care, rather than feeling threatened by focusing on what is problematic.

This type of inquiry and learning, based on and in one's own practice, is often termed 'active learning'.

Practice pointer 4.5

Developing a person-centred learning culture requires processes that enable individuals and teams to consider their own and their organization's beliefs, values, behaviours and systems, and whether they are consistent with person-centred values.

Activity 4.3

What might hinder your team from wanting to engage in exploring the person-centredness of their practice? What might help to overcome this?

Active learning

The term 'active learning' is often linked with the kind of learning that is required to develop practice. It could be argued that any learning that requires engagement by and effort from those involved is active (Dewing 2010). However, active learning in the context of practice development methodology means that people do not just participate in thinking and analysing information, but centre this on practice. In addition, the practice in question is their own practice, and the exploration and analysis is focused on this and consideration of how it can be developed (Dewing 2008, 2010, McCormack et al. 2009). People's learning is not just linked to their work, but arises from this, the individuals themselves, the people they work with and their particular circumstances (McCormack et al. 2009, Dewing 2010). For Sahib, this point is important, because he thinks that in order to develop a more person-centred approach to care, his team need to actively engage in exploring how they practise, day to day. This includes what drives their practice, both within themselves and in their environment, and what this may mean in terms of whether or not the care they provide is person centred. These principles are congruent with what Sahib knows about practice development methodology, where the people involved, including patients and practitioners, and the context of practice are key to understanding what happens and why it happens (Manley et al. 2009, Finset 2011).

Practice pointer 4.6

Active learning:

• occurs when individuals think about, explore and analyse information centred on their own practice, and use this to consider how their practice can be developed
• arises from individuals themselves and their work, colleagues and workplace.

Because active learning is based on real, specific events that happen in a particular context, it makes use of all the sources and types of information that are relevant to the situation in question. Chapter 6 discusses the types of evidence that can be useful in developing person-centred practice, but developing a person-centred learning culture focuses on exploring the values, beliefs, perspectives and interpretations of reality of all the people concerned, and the tacit knowledge gained from practice situations (Dewing 2008, 2010, McCormack et al. 2009). This is consistent with the principles of critical social theory and critical realism, which underpin practice development methodology. These perspectives view people's personal knowledge, values and perceptions, the power that individuals and groups have, or see themselves as having, and what makes people interpret things as they do as crucial to understanding situations (Freeman and Vasconcelos 2010, Bevan et al. 2012, Lapum et al. 2012, Oliver 2012). In addition, they see the history, as well as the current situation, of individuals and organizations as vital to gaining insight into what they are and how they practise (Freeman and Vasconcelos 2010).

Sahib thinks that using active learning techniques will be instrumental to his team developing person-centred care. For person-centredness to become the driving force in care provision, it will need to be something people want to achieve and see as a real possibility in their workplace. The types of knowledge that will be critical to achieving this will be those that enable people to understand what makes them believe what they do about themselves, the people with whom they work and their workplace, and how this influences their actions. Without developing this personal knowledge, any changes in practice that happen are likely to be relatively superficial and behavioural, rather than based on a genuine transformation of how people see their work and want to practise.

Practice pointer 4.7

The information used in active learning can include:

- learning from oneself
- learning from colleagues
- learning from patients and their relatives.

Practice pointer 4.8

The knowledge used to inform active learning may include:

- values, beliefs and priorities
- personal perspectives and interpretations
- tacit knowledge gained from practice situations.

An important outcome of active learning for Sahib is that it should directly influence practice (McCormack et al. 2009). He thinks it will be comparatively easy for people to discuss the importance of person-centredness and agree that this would be a good way to work. He doubts if many of his team will oppose this as an ideal. However, without applying it to the complexities of their own practice and exploring what aids and inhibits it, he thinks it could easily remain a pleasing ideal, which will not necessarily influence their day-to-day work a great deal. He hopes that by actively exploring the person-centredness of their own practice, individuals will be enabled to positively challenge their mindsets and the ethos and culture of their team and workplace. This links with the philosophical underpinnings of practice development methodology, where the emancipation and transformation of individuals and workplaces are key goals (Dewing 2010). Exploring person-centredness in terms of their own day-to-day practice may enable individuals and the team as a whole to feel and think differently about their work and, as a result, transform how they approach people and situations (Dewing 2008, 2010). It may also mean that they feel empowered to do things they intrinsically think are right but currently feel inhibited from doing.

An additional benefit that Sahib has identified from this approach to learning is that if the team's beliefs, values and ways of working are jointly challenged, the cultural expectation may become that the right thing to do is the person-centred thing. The team's goals will then be able to legitimately and openly move from being, for example, to enable patients to comply with what professionals see as beneficial, to enabling what matters to patients to direct the care they receive. As Chapter 3 identified, this will involve some degree of risk, but by becoming a team expectation, this may enable it to be discussed, and individuals to be supported in working in this way.

A key factor in active learning, however, is not just the learning that takes place at a particular point in time, but that those involved learn how the process of learning in and from practice works, and continue this process (McCormack et al. 2009). Achieving a culture in which this type of learning is the norm often requires facilitation to enable individuals and teams to gain the skills and confidence to develop and continue their own reflective inquiries within and about their practice (van der Zijpp and Dowling 2009).

Activity 4.4

What might affect you or your team achieving person-centred care? Think of the values, beliefs, personal perspectives, interpretations and knowledge of yourself, your colleagues, your organization and those for whom you care.

Practice pointer 4.9

Active learning includes practitioners learning how the process of learning in and from practice works, so that it is continuous and not a one-off occurrence.

Facilitation of reflection

Active learning may require people to think and learn in an unfamiliar way. So, especially in the early stages, it can be useful to have someone who is experienced in facilitating this approach to work with individuals and groups to enable them to develop their skills and confidence (Dewing 2010). Sahib and his team are all familiar with supervision, reflection and debriefing processes, as these are commonly used in practice. Sahib is used to taking a lead role in exploring situations that have occurred with the team and in facilitating reflection on incidents or concerns. However, he thinks that the type of reflection that will be needed to develop a more person-centred approach to practice, with its focus on supportively challenging the present ethos of care, will be slightly different. It therefore seems to him that it will be beneficial for the team to employ the services of an external facilitator to work with them on learning to use this approach to develop person-centred care. Employing the services of an external facilitator also means that he will be a co-participant in the process of exploration and questioning, not a manager in a position of authority, who might be perceived to be criticizing the care the team currently provides.

The facilitation of active learning involves enabling people to engage in challenging what they take for granted. In this case, Sahib thinks it will be necessary to challenge what he and his team assume to be the right way to approach care, the ideal outcomes of care and the best way to interact with patients. The skills required to achieve this type of exploration include active listening, noticing what is said but also what is not said, asking oneself and others a range of purposeful questions, giving feedback, and actively seeking and receiving feedback from others (Titchen et al. 2013). The intention of these processes is to enable those who are engaged in learning to uncover new ways of seeing things.

Practice pointer 4.10

Active learning involves:

- challenging what is taken for granted
- actively listening to oneself and others
- noticing what is said and what is not said
- asking oneself and others a range of focused questions
- giving, receiving and requesting feedback.

The process of critical reflection is one of the key tools practice development methodology uses to enable individuals and groups to develop insights into their practice (Peek et al. 2007, Dewing 2010, Brown and McCormack 2011). This process requires people to be able to think retrospectively and critically about particular practice events, what affected them, and how things could have been, had particular elements of the situation been handled differently. It includes people considering what the desired outcomes of a situation were, what the actual outcomes were, what match or mismatch occurred, and what caused this to be the case. This can include examining individual and group perceptions, and the meanings that are attributed to situations (Dewing 2010). In terms of developing person-centredness, it also involves identifying what, within individuals, teams and organizations, in a given situation, did or did not enable person-centred practice to occur.

Reflection can be achieved by using established models of reflection, or more individual and creative approaches (Dewing 2010). No one approach is right or best: this will depend on the team and individuals concerned, and the situation in question. The key point is that reflection aimed at assisting in developing person-centred practice has to move beyond exploring the superficial to examining the in-depth (McCormack et al. 2009, Manley et al. 2009, Brown and McCormack 2011). This includes engagement in the process of considering exactly what causes people to act, or not act, in the way that they do, and requires individuals to listen carefully to themselves and others (Brown and McCormack 2011).

As Chapter 2 identified, the theories on which practice development methodology draws include critical realism and critical social theory. These theories view the reasons for perceptions and events as being a complex combination not just of the present, but also of the history, culture and context in which they occur (Freeman and Vasconcelos 2010, Bevan et al. 2012, Lapum et al. 2012). Well-facilitated critical reflection should therefore enable people to explore how complex interlinking factors from the present and past, and hopes for the future, influence individual and corporate perceptions, behaviours and practice. High-quality critical reflection, like the critical creativity seen in practice development methodology, also requires some degree of creative imagining so that a vision of what things could be like can be developed (Dewing 2010, Manley et al. 2013a).

The idea of using this type of critical reflection appeals to Sahib. He thinks that his team's experience in reflecting on practice situations will enable them to build on a familiar concept, but to develop this to explore their perceptions, values, priorities, beliefs, what influences these, and how they can creatively develop more person-centred ways of working. He is, however, mindful of his intention to underpin this journey into person-centredness with the principles of appreciative inquiry. It is important to Sahib that his team see this process as encouragement to further develop what is good about their work. Despite supportively challenging what people do and what directs their work, he believes that it will be important to emphasize the positive aspects of existing practice throughout the process; for example, by focusing on instances where people have acted in a person-centred way and what enabled this to happen, as well as what could be improved.

Practice development methodology pays great attention to practitioners becoming capable of facilitating learning in themselves and others (Larsen et al. 2005, Manley et al. 2013b). It therefore aims to enable individuals not only to gain insights into their practice, but also to understand how they gained these insights, so that they become able to facilitate their own learning and that of their colleagues (Dewing 2010). Sahib sees this as important for his team. Given that funding for external facilitation will be finite, his team, individually and as a group, need to become able to challenge themselves and their own practice, day to day, so that any developments they make are sustained and taken further. It is, nonetheless, often valuable for someone to be available to continue to facilitate individual and team reflection (Newman et al. 2009). Sahib thinks that over time, as the team become more adept in using active learning processes themselves, their external facilitators' input will reduce. However, he believes that having some ongoing external facilitation will always be useful to help to sustain the impetus for practice-based, person-centred learning, and he will therefore need to make a case for the resources to support this.

Practice pointer 4.11

In critical reflection, individuals think retrospectively, critically and in depth about:

- what the desired outcomes of a situation were
- what the actual outcomes were
- what match or mismatch occurred
- what contributed to this being the case.

In practice development methodology, this includes identifying what, within individuals, teams and organizations, did or did not enable person-centred practice to happen.

Activity 4.5

Think of a particular practice event where you or a colleague acted in a person-centred way. What enabled this to happen?

High challenge/high support

A key part of the facilitation of effective practice-based reflective learning is using high challenge/high support techniques (McCormack et al. 2009, Manley et al. 2009, Titchen et al. 2013). Here, the intention is to challenge and support people in reflecting critically on their practice. In this approach, a facilitator usually works alongside an individual, challenging their everyday assumptions about practice and supporting them to look at the reasons for successes and alternatives to areas where things have not gone so well. This 'critical companionship' means that someone in the situation with the individual supportively challenges what is automatically done or is assumed to be a good way of working (Manley et al. 2013b). The intention of this process is to help people become aware of taken-for-granted assumptions about aspects of their practice and have the opportunity to explore different ways of viewing the world (Wilson et al. 2006, Manley et al. 2009). The advantage of having a facilitator working closely with individuals in everyday practice is that it enables attention to be brought to the subconscious actions, expressions or messages they engage in or convey to others (Wilson et al. 2006). These may be positive or things that could be improved, but highlighting them enables the person concerned to develop, replicate or try to modify them. The process is termed 'high challenge/high support', because it has to include support, so that people feel empowered, and not destroyed, by the challenges they are presented with.

Sahib thinks that this kind of critical companionship will be valuable in developing a culture of active, person-centred learning. However, as his team mainly work in people's homes, on-the-spot reflection with a facilitator may be difficult. He does, however, think that it might be adapted to practitioners engaging in discussions with a facilitator immediately after individual visits.

Practice pointer 4.12

Critical companionship and high challenge/high support methods can enable assumptions about practice to be challenged, while also supporting individuals to look at the reasons for successes and alternatives to areas where there is less success.

While developing the skills of critical reflection is an important part of developing practice, this does not automatically lead to reflexive practice, which is seen as a key part of person-centred care. Reflexivity is defined as having an ongoing conversation (often with oneself) about an experience while living in the moment. It involves questioning what influences a given situation in real time by standing back from the experience and considering the values, beliefs, priorities, structures and understandings of the situation that are affecting what is happening (Brown and McCormack 2011). It draws on the thinking and reflective skills seen in critical reflection, but is more immediate and relates directly to what is happening at a given moment in time. Sahib thinks that having someone to act as a critical companion for his team may enable them to begin to learn and embed the skills of reflexive, person-centred thinking in their day-to-day work (Manley et al. 2009).

Practice pointer 4.13

Reflexivity is a process of standing back from and analysing a situation while being actively involved in it. It includes considering the values, beliefs, priorities, structures and perceptions of the situation that are influencing what happens.

Individuals developing the skills of reflection and reflexivity and being able to engage in giving and receiving feedback that challenges the status quo are all important parts of altering workplace cultures (Dewing 2010). However, Dewing (2010) suggests that developing the skills of personal reflection generally needs to precede reflective dialogue with colleagues. People may need to develop their skills in exploring and challenging their own feelings and thoughts before being able to confidently offer real challenges to the views or actions of others. Thus, facilitators often need to work with individuals, and subsequently with groups, on developing the skills of critical reflection.

To this end, Sahib initially plans to hold a meeting with his whole team to discuss his ideas and gain their perspectives. He intends to follow this by individuals working one to one with a facilitator to begin to reflect on the person-centredness of their work. This will precede, and then become a part of, an ongoing system of one-to-one high challenge/high support working and reflective group dialogues related to how the team can develop and sustain person-centred practice.

Reflective dialogue and creative approaches

Sahib's intention is for the exploration of the team's ethos and values to be conducted in a challenging but supportive and positive way. His team are, in many respects, experienced and skilled communicators, but a part of their learning may concern how to challenge each other meaningfully but support-ively and communicate effectively in relation to developing person-centred practice (Dewing 2010). In addition, as Chan (2013) identifies, they may not all consider becoming critically creative in their thinking and practice desira-ble or a priority.

The dialogue people engage in will need to be nonjudgmental and cooper-ative, with positive language and time for people to listen attentively, reflect, respond and engage in collaborative learning and creative imagining (Walsh et al. 2009, Dewing 2010). This sort of conversation is not always the norm in workplaces, particularly where services are busy and staff under pressure. Even where it is the intention, the opportunity and time to develop such discussions can be more difficult to achieve than is often supposed (Walsh et al. 2009, Boomer and McCormack 2010, Dewing 2010). Sahib is aware that his team are busy, and because they work in people's homes, they do not often have a great deal of time together. They tend to get on well as a team and support each other at difficult times, but there is often simply not enough time for them to be together and engage in any depth of conversation. Even debriefing after particular events is often largely based around reassuring one another that, despite the odds, they did the best they could. As Albarran (2004) highlights, a challenge for Sahib will be to create the time and space for his team to be able to spend time listening to themselves and each other and think creatively about their practice.

Sahib thinks that gaining the services of an outside facilitator will effec-tively give staff permission to take the time to engage in critically reflective and creative thinking. He also believes that expert facilitation may be necessary to enable the team to develop their creative thinking skills, become open to new interpretations of events, and develop innovative ways of working (Albarran 2004). In addition, such facilitation may be a means of providing opportuni-ties for the team to develop their creative thinking through approaches they might not otherwise consider or feel confident to use, such as arts media or creative writing (McCormack and Titchen 2006).

Activity 4.6

What would be the benefits of your team using critically reflective processes? What would the challenges be and how might these be overcome?

Practice pointer 4.14

Creating the time and space to reflect and an ethos in which this is seen as a valid use of time are essential to developing person-centred reflection.

Summary

Sahib recognizes that a key part of developing person-centred care will be for individuals and his team as a whole to engage in real-time, practice-based learning. This will require them to develop and continue to hone the skills of critically creative, reflective and reflexive working, as individuals and as a group. To achieve this, Sahib plans to access the services of an external facilitator who can work with his team on creating and sustaining a culture in which ongoing reflective and reflexive learning becomes a habit rather than a task. His intention is for this to include the use of high challenge/high support approaches, within an ethos of appreciative inquiry, in which the positive attributes and talents of individuals and the team as a whole, rather than their deficits, lead the process.

Sahib is, at the same time, mindful that to really achieve person-centred care, patients have to be central to the process of developing practice. He is now planning to explore how he can incorporate patients into this process.

Case scenario

Kerry is the senior sister of an outpatients department. Although the department generally meets waiting time targets and has a harmonious atmosphere, there have been some complaints recently that patients feel they are part of a conveyor belt of care. Kerry wants to explore how the team could develop a more person-centred approach to working, but also sees the department as having many positive attributes, and does not want this exploration to detract from the team's strengths. So, she intends to begin by looking at what her team do well, rather than what needs to improve.

What Kerry's team do well

Kerry thinks her team run a professional, efficient service. They work well as a team, and collaborate effectively with a number of other disciplines and departments to make the service run as it should, even when it is busy. Her team strive to meet waiting targets, and make a point of keeping patients up to date regarding delays or unexpected changes in plans. The different disciplines involved are generally respectful of and good humoured with one another. The department has considerably expanded its activities over recent years, so that patients have less visits, or less locations to visit, within the hospital. As well as seeing medical staff, patients can be seen by physiother- apists, occupational therapists and clinical nurse specialists, and can have a range of long-term care needs assessed and managed. The team are generally keen to improve their practice, actively seek patient feedback, and try to act on suggestions for improving the service they provide.

Kerry feels that her team have many strengths, including a genuine desire to offer a good quality service, which could be used to help them to develop a more person-centred approach to their work.

How could Kerry use her team's strengths to develop a more person-centred approach to care?

Kerry's team are usually receptive to ideas and ready to question what they do. They are committed to providing good care and try to see things from the patient's perspective. They are almost universally courteous to patients, even in challenging circumstances, and try to resolve any difficulties that arise with them. This all leads her to believe that they would probably be receptive to the idea of trying to make care more person centred.

The team also strive to work well with their colleagues. As well as being amenable to developing person-centred care from the perspective of patients, Kerry considers it likely that they will have a mindset that enables them to want to adopt an approach in which staff, as well as patients, are seen as people.

Kerry feels positive about the possibility of her team being able to use their strengths to adopt a more person-centred approach to working. However, there are also some things she thinks might inhibit this.

What might hinder Kerry's team from wanting to engage in exploring the person-centredness of their practice? What might help to overcome this?

Kerry's team are committed to providing a high standard of care, but she thinks it could be challenging and threatening for them to have to question the person-centredness of their care. It might also be disheartening for them, because they currently perceive that they provide good care, with limited resources.

Kerry thinks that by focusing on the team's many strengths, she may be able to encourage them to see developing care to be more person centred as the next step in developing existing good practice, not a dismissal of all their hard work and what they have achieved. She feels that by emphasizing that the aim is to build on their strengths, she may be able to introduce this as a positive, non-threatening idea.

While she wants to introduce the idea of developing person-centred practice as a positive thing, Kerry also thinks there will be factors within individuals and the team as a whole that might stand in the way of this being achieved.

What might affect Kerry's team achieving person-centred care?

Personal and team values and beliefs: Kerry and her team value providing an efficient service. Becoming person, rather than service, centred carries the risk that the way appointments are made or people dealt with on arrival and during appointments will be less predictable and therefore less efficient.

Personal and team perspectives: Kerry and her team perceive that things work well in the department because they have systems in place that keep things running smoothly, and into which people, including patients and staff, slot efficiently. The department is commonly described as a 'tightly run ship' and this is its key strength in many people's view. People on Kerry's team may be concerned that being more person centred will challenge this, because an individual's particular needs or preferences may be difficult to accommodate and meeting them may lead to a less efficient use of scarce time and resources.

Personal knowledge: Kerry knows that she likes to be in control of her work, and can find it threatening to move away from what is quite a regimented approach to how things are done. While she sees being more person centred as desirable, she still wants the outpatients department to run smoothly. In addition, Kerry knows that her colleagues and the organization as a whole will view any move away from their current reputation as caring, but efficient, negatively, despite the adverse comments that have led her to review service provision.

Patient perspectives: The people who use the outpatients department will probably not want a less efficient service. They often comment on the value of knowing they will be seen on time, or told of any delays. Although the department has received occasional comments that it is like a conveyor belt, Kerry's team have always considered this to be an accepted and necessary compromise in order to secure timely and efficient services.

Kerry thinks that, for herself and others, it will be useful to think of instances where working in a person-centred way has not compromised what the department and those who use it value.

A particular practice event where one of Kerry's colleagues acted in a person-centred way and what enabled this to happen

Kerry recalled a recent event where Mr Hammond, who attends the department for a number of reasons, came in to have his leg ulcer wounds assessed. Mr Hammond lives in a nursing home and the carer who brings him in is never able to stay with him, despite negotiations between the department and nursing home about this. During his early visits, Mr Hammond became rather agitated while he waited, so a member of staff is now allocated to keep an eye on him and the receptionist chats to him when she can. With frequent visits from staff and reminders of when and why he will be seen, Mr Hammond is now usually fairly calm during his visits.

On his last but one visit the person who was allocated to keep an eye on Mr Hammond asked him about where he had lived before his current location. He told her about his house, his family and his previous job. He had worked as a head engineer in large aerospace company and told her a little about the work he had done. Before he had finished talking to her, it was time for his appointment.

Initially, Kerry's colleague wondered if she had left others with an unreasonable workload while she chatted to Mr Hammond. However, the general feeling was that it had been useful for her to focus on Mr Hammond. It had made him calmer, both while waiting and during his appointment. Knowing Mr Hammond's story also caused other people in the department to think more about him as a person with a history, rather than as a problem that needed to be managed efficiently. Kerry thought about how difficult it must be for a person who had held a managerial role in a large company to be in his situation. She came across some magazines about the air industry, which she brought in for Mr Hammond's next appointment. He sat leafing through them while he waited, and although a member of staff again made themself available to talk to him, he seemed quite content reading the magazines.

What enabled this to happen, in Kerry's view, was that a member of staff was prepared to take the risk of doing something differently. She began her dialogue by focusing on Mr Hammond, and who he was, not on the service he had attended for. She did not tell him about what he was there for or how long he would wait, but engaged with him. She was also part of a team who would be likely to respect her decision, but also to challenge it if necessary, which gave her the confidence to do this.

This was an example of how person-centred working enhanced care provision, but also enabled the department to continue to run efficiently by drawing on the team working, care and respect for one another they already had.

Kerry felt that she could use Mr Hammond's story to introduce the idea of critical reflection that focused on positive, rather than negative, experiences to enable the team to develop more person-centred care.

What would be the benefits of Kerry's team using critically reflective processes?

Kerry thought that the benefits of using critically reflective processes would be that people would be able to see how their personal and team practice could be developed to be more person centred, without sacrificing what mattered to them. It might also enable them to review what did matter to them. This would allow them to understand how what they did well could be enhanced or used to develop other areas of practice, and how what they struggled with could be addressed. It would mean that they had the chance to see things they had not seen before or had taken for granted, including positive elements of their work that had gone unnoticed as a part of standard practice.

Embedding this process in their everyday work would mean that, over time, it became an automatic part of what the team did and a part of, not a challenge to, the effective running of the department.

What would be the challenges, and how might they be overcome?

One of the challenges that Kerry's team might encounter concerned whether the team felt confident in critically reflecting on their practice. This might be overcome by employing the services of an experienced and skilled facilitator to work initially one to one with individuals, and then engage them in group discussions.

Additional challenges were time and resources. These included not just the time for reflective sessions, but also arranging these so that part-time staff could participate. Kerry thought this might be helped by a facilitator initially engaging in one-to-one work with individuals, which would be flexible for those working part-time hours. For group sessions, she would need to plan carefully so that everyone could participate. This might involve discussions about how they would ensure that even if not everyone could attend every session, over time everyone had opportunities to participate.

Funding for procuring a facilitator's time might be a challenge, and would need to be taken from the budget for staff development. However, person-centred care was high on the trust agenda and Kerry could link this to the complaints that had been received about the department being seen as a conveyor belt system. Thus, although she wanted to maintain a focus on the positives of the department, the problems that had been encountered might have to be highlighted in order to secure funding.

Additional resources

Appreciative inquiry
www.mindtools.com/pages/article/newTMC_85.htm
Describes what appreciative inquiry is and how it can be used.

http://appreciativeinquiry.case.edu
A portal devoted to the sharing of resources and tools related to appreciative inquiry.

http://centerforappreciativeinquiry.net
Center for Appreciative Inquiry, with links to resources about appreciative inquiry.

Developing person-centred cultures
www.pcpmn.cswebsites.org/Libraries/Local/805/Docs/Microsoft%20Word%20
-%20Person%20Centred%20Culture.pdf
A report on the process of working towards a person-centred culture.

www.nds.org.au/asset/view_document/979319712
A guide on developing and implementing person-centred approaches.

Critical reflection
www.mcgraw-hill.co.uk/openup/chapters/0335218784.pdf
A chapter on critical reflection.

www.education.vic.gov.au/Documents/childhood/professionals/support/reffram.pdf
Information about what critical reflection is and how it works.

5 Developing Practice in Partnership with Patients

Chapter overview

- Practice development methodology aims to develop practice in a way that keeps patients and their particular and individual needs central. This logically means that patients should play a key part in every stage of the practice development process.
- Engaging patients in practice development processes should allow meaningful dialogue to take place concerning what should, and can, be done to enable person-centred practice to develop.
- Key issues to consider in involving patients in developing practice are: what the intention of their involvement is, who to involve, how to involve them, what preparation people will need for working together, and how the value of participation will be clear to patients, practitioners and organizations.

Sarah is the senior sister of an intensive care unit (ICU). The nurses who work on the unit are seeking to develop a more person-centred way of working and intend to use the principles of practice development methodology to achieve this. They have identified that patients should be a central part of the process of developing practice, and therefore want to include them in their practice development work. Sarah's team have considered how they might be able to achieve this, and, because of the acuity of illness of those who are cared for on ICUs, have concluded that they will need to invite ex-patients to be involved. However, before proceeding further, they want to be sure that they approach incorporating people who have been patients in their practice development activities in a way that makes their involvement a real and central part of the process.

> **Practice pointer 5.1**
>
> Practice development methodology places patients at the centre of care, making it logical for them to be involved in the process of developing practice.

Integrating patients into practice development processes

The ethos of practice development methodology is person-centredness: it focuses on the people who receive care, and aims to develop practice in a way that keeps them and their particular and individual needs central (McCormack et al. 2009). This means that those people should be a key part of every stage of developing practice, so that developments are beneficial to them, as perceived by them (McCormack et al. 2006). This is the ethos that Sarah's team subscribes to. They know about the technical and medical aspects of care, and can possibly imagine what might matter to people who are patients in an ICU, or people visiting a relative in an ICU. However, they cannot fully appreciate what it would be like to be a patient in an ICU, and what would matter most to individuals in that situation. The ICU staff have a number of ideas about visiting, noise, lighting, continuity of care, privacy, talking to patients and having personal effects available that might enhance care provision. However, they recognize that they are essentially second-guessing what is important to patients in an ICU and what makes a difference to them. Most importantly, they want to explore what would make people feel that their personhood (as discussed in Chapter 3) is respected in the ICU, and how they, as a team, can work towards achieving this.

As well as focusing on personhood, practice development methodology draws on the principles of critical social theory and critical realism, which both emphasize power issues and their effect on how individuals and groups function (Freeman and Vasconcelos 2010, Bevan et al. 2012, Lapum et al. 2012, Parlour and McCormack 2012). Involving patients in developments in healthcare is consistent with the aim of empowering them, but differs from how they were historically viewed, as passive and subservient recipients of care designed and provided by professionals (Braye and Preston-Shoot 2005, Bradshaw 2008, Higgins et al. 2011). In contrast, integrating patients into the process of developing services places them as consumers of healthcare, whose opinions should be sought, listened to and acted upon (O'Boyle-Duggan and Gretch 2012, Tong et al. 2012, Ward et al. 2013).

Sarah and her team see enabling ex-ICU patients to influence practice as important, but potentially challenging. Patients in ICUs are usually acutely critically ill, highly reliant on staff, and generally have limited communication options, which is likely to make their ICU stay a disempowering experience.

These feelings of disempowerment may persist even after people are discharged from the ICU, particularly when they are in contact with the professionals who cared for them during their ICU stay. Their perceptions of their role while in the ICU, along with an often-expressed gratitude to staff for their physical recovery, may make enabling them to challenge existing service provision difficult. When Sarah has sought informal feedback from ex-patients in the past, she has found that people tend to be uncomfortable about making critical comments about the care they received. However, she also knows from the literature that being a patient in an ICU can be a negative experience. Sarah's team want ex-patients to work with them as equal partners in sharing experiences and developing services, but they are aware that this may be easier for them to want than achieve. Sarah thinks that the focus of practice development methodology on learning, individually and as a team, to reflect and supportively and nonjudgmentally challenge the status quo will be useful in this respect (McCormack et al. 2006, Wilson and McCormack 2006). She hopes that if ex-patients can engage with the ICU team in processes of critical reflection, such as those described in Chapter 4, they will develop their ability and confidence to contribute to discussions about how practice could become more person centred.

Sarah and her team have, however, also considered what involving patients really means and what it will look like in practice.

Activity 5.1

What might contribute to the patients you care for feeling disempowered?

Practice pointer 5.2

- Involving patients in developing practice is consistent with the ethos of patient empowerment seen in practice development methodology.
- Meaningfully involving patients in developing practice places them as equal partners whose voice should be heard and acted on.
- This differs from the historic view of patients as passive and subservient recipients of care.

What is patient involvement?

Sarah and her colleagues have come across a range approaches for involving patients in healthcare developments. These span peripheral involvement, such as a one-off consultation at one end of the continuum, through to patients being involved in every stage of the process and taking the majority of control in how services develop, at the other (Smith et al. 2008). These levels of involvement are often linked with how far the process of being involved in developing practice empowers patients, with the highest degrees of empowerment occurring when patients adopt key roles in determining what should be available, deciding how this should be provided, agreeing how resources should be used, and evaluating services (Smith et al. 2008, Tritter 2009). There is, however, no one best way to involve patients in developing practice: the best approach depends on the situation in question, the people involved, and the rationale for their involvement (Armstrong et al. 2013). A whole process approach to patient involvement is what Sarah's team aspire to, with ex-patients being a part of suggesting, designing, directing and evaluating developments (Dewing et al. 2006, Cotterell et al. 2010, Rose et al. 2010).

Practice pointer 5.3

Patients can be involved in developing practice at different levels including:

* a one-off consultation
* occasional consultations
* involvement in some parts of the process
* full integration in the whole process, including decision making at the design, enactment and evaluation stages.

Sarah and her team want to use terminology that accurately reflects what they aim to achieve, so that there is a clear and shared understanding of the intention of including ex-patients in the process of developing practice (Rise et al. 2013). They have discovered that the terms used to describe what might be broadly termed 'patient involvement' are not consistent (Borg et al. 2009, Tritter 2009). These terms, which seem to be used somewhat interchangeably, include involvement, engagement, participation, gaining perspectives, empowerment, collaboration, and partnership (Borg et al. 2009, Tritter 2009). However, these seem to Sarah to refer to slightly different ideas about the intention, focus, practicalities and outcomes of patients being a part of developments in care provision (Borg et al. 2009).

The terms 'participation' and 'involvement' suggest less influence than 'empowerment', and may encompass a range of levels of participation or involvement from minimal through to real engagement in all parts of the process of developing practice (Borg et al. 2009). Empowerment is something that Sarah and her team hope to achieve through their practice development activities, but empowering ex-patients is not the core intended focus of their activities. The aim of their practice development processes is not only to empower patients, but also to achieve person-centredness. Person-centredness involves regarding everyone as a person and, as Chapter 2 highlighted, this means practitioners as well as patients being seen as people, who may, for a variety of reasons, feel unable to question or develop the way they work. Disempowered staff may also struggle to empower patients, or be intimidated by empowered patients (King and Kelly 2011). Practice development methodology acknowledges that practitioners as well as patients need to be empowered, and Sarah's team want to base their work with ex-patients on the principles of equality and mutual respect, not unequal power belonging to, or being developed by, any party.

Practice pointer 5.4

Terms that can be used to describe patients being a part of developing practice include involvement, participation, gaining perspectives, inclusion, empowerment, collaboration, engagement and partnership. The term used in any given situation should accurately reflect the intention of the activities concerned.

The key aim of Sarah's team in working with ex-patients is to achieve a mutual understanding of one another's perspectives, and to use this to develop practice in ways that will be beneficial for patients but also achievable for staff. This will require open, honest and respectful dialogue, in which each party shares their knowledge and perspectives and listens to and takes on board those of others (Rise et al. 2013). This suggests to Sarah that a partnership approach, with equality of status, power and respect, will be needed (Rise et al. 2013). To achieve this, practitioners and ex-patients will need to be involved jointly, meaningfully and consistently throughout the process of developing practice. This will require time and resources, so Sarah wants to formally identify what the benefits of working in partnership with ex-patients are likely to be, in order to justify these.

Activity 5.2

If you were to involve patients in developments in practice, what would your intention be? What term would you use to describe this?

Practice pointer 5.5

Patients should be involved in practice development partnerships that are:

- meaningful
- congruent with the intentions of their involvement
- clear, honest and transparent.

Benefits of working in partnership with patients

One argument for involving patients in developments in practice is not so much that it is beneficial but that it is right, as they are the key stakeholders in health services and therefore entitled to influence them (Armstrong et al. 2013). They are probably the most able to say whether proposed developments in practice are likely to improve things for, or matter to, those receiving care. This will, in turn, enable professionals to direct time and resources to achieving improvements that will be meaningful for the recipients of services (Braye and Preston-Shoot 2005, Hoole and Morgan 2010, Diaz del Campo et al. 2011, Tong et al. 2012, Ward et al. 2013). Equally, if real sharing and partnership are achieved, patients will gain a better insight into what professionals perceive as important and why this is so, which may enhance their understanding and thus their experience of care.

Involving patients in the whole process of developing practice can also assist in maintaining the momentum for change and ensuring that promised improvements materialize and are sustained (Evans et al. 2013). This can include not just whether promised developments happen, but whether they develop in the way that patients wanted, expected or think will be useful. Sarah considers this a key issue, because, even with good intentions, it is often possible for proposed developments to be sidetracked or change slightly as things progress. Having ex-patients on board throughout the process of developing practice is likely to be a useful guard against this happening. However, she is also aware that, for this to be seen as beneficial, all levels of staff need to be committed to the value of working in partnership with patients. If not, patients holding the process of developing practice to account could be seen as a threat, or downside, of their involvement, rather than an advantage.

The existence of effective practice development partnerships with patients can improve people's confidence in contributing to healthcare development processes (Evans et al. 2013). If patients feel that their involvement is meaningful and has real outcomes, they may be more willing to make the time and effort to continue to be involved, and encourage others to do so. Conversely, if they see their involvement as tokenistic, with no real effect, they are less likely to continue to participate, or encourage others to do so (Beresford 2010, Rose et al. 2010).

Practice pointer 5.6

- Patient involvement can be beneficial for staff, organizations and current and future patients.
- Patient involvement in the whole process of practice development can help to sustain and extend developments over time.

These benefits seem to Sarah to be a valid justification of the resources that will be required to work in partnership with ex-patients to develop person-centred practice. Nonetheless, one of the challenges of articulating the value of integrating patients into the process of developing practice is that it is unlikely to produce measurable outcomes, especially in the short term (Evans et al. 2013). Sarah does not believe that working in partnership with ex-patients to develop person-centred care will be able to be directly linked to immediate and measurable changes in outcomes for ICU patients. This is something that she thinks requires clarity from the outset: the intention of working in partnership with ex-patients is not to improve measurable outcomes. Rather, it is intended to contribute to developing a more person-centred approach to care provision, and it is against this aim that its success or otherwise should to be judged. As well as individuals within the ICU buying into this concept, Sarah is aware that more senior managers need to see this as a valid outcome. The development of person-centred care is currently a priority in her organization, but will have to continue to be viewed as an important outcome in its own right for the necessary resources to be made available for it to become, and remain, a reality.

In order to be clear about what resources they will need, and when they will need them, Sarah and her team are considering the practical steps that will be required for them to achieve partnership working with ex-ICU patients. They think they need to begin the process by enabling everyone concerned to understand the rationale for seeking to work in partnership with ex-patients.

Activity 5.3

What would the advantages and challenges be in involving patients in developing practice in your workplace?

Rationale for working in partnership with patients

Sarah thinks that the rationale for the ICU team working in partnership with ex-patients to develop practice needs to be clear from the beginning and understood by all those involved in the process (Braye and Preston-Shoot 2005, Rose et al. 2010, Tong et al. 2012, Armstrong et al. 2013). The resources needed to develop practice include time and adequate staffing for meetings and discussions to clarify the reason for, and aims of, this approach to developing practice.

Sarah and her team's main rationale for involving ex-patients is that they will know what mattered most to them during their stay in the ICU and what affected their perceptions of the quality of their care. They also hope that it will enable practitioners to better appreciate patients as people and use this to achieve person-centredness in care. There may be other desirable and specific outcomes, such as improving visiting arrangements or reducing night-time disturbances for patients, but these are not the focus of the process of developing practice. These key reasons for involving ex-patients in developing practice mean that it is necessary to involve them as soon as possible in the process, which may be important for Sarah to clarify when seeking resources. The rationale is also important in terms of how the process of involvement is managed, starting with who should be involved and how they will be found.

Who to involve

Although person-centredness recognizes that patients are not one homogeneous group, every patient who has ever been admitted to an ICU will not, realistically, be able to be invited to participate in the proposed practice development activities. Thus, Sarah and her team need to use some kind of invitation or selection process.

Gaining meaningful representation from patients requires decisions about who to involve and how to recruit them (Armstrong et al. 2013). For Sarah's team, this includes considering whether the people concerned simply need to have experienced being a patient on an ICU, be representative of particular demographic characteristics of the population of ICU patients (such as age group, gender, reason for admission), or whether they need to have particular skills and capabilities. Their reason for involving ex-patients forms a useful guide for making these decisions (Armstrong et al. 2013). Their rationale is to enable patient perspectives to drive the development of person-centred care. As such, Sarah thinks that it may be important to have input from people who were admitted to an ICU for different reasons, including planned surgery that was expected to include a stay in an ICU, emergency admissions, long-term stays and short stays, as these might create different experiences. She also believes that it could be useful for different age groups and genders to be represented. Nonetheless, because the key aim is for people to share their individual perspectives of having been an ICU patient, she sees these as considerations, not absolute requirements, in deciding who to invite to participate in the process. As the intention is to develop person-centred care, rather than particular aspects of practice, she does not think that any specific skills or knowledge will be necessary, other than the knowledge gained from having been a patient on an ICU.

The next challenge for Sarah's team is to decide how to recruit ex-patients. They could do this by asking for volunteers, issuing invitations to specific people, or seeking advice from others about who to invite to participate. There are pros and cons to each approach. Sarah's team choosing the people to approach might mean that those with specific skills, knowledge or experiences can be targeted. They could, for example, invite people who they know will speak their minds, not be intimidated, but also act respectfully to others.

There are two ex-ICU patients who Sarah knows are involved in other initiatives within the NHS trust, and are used to acting as patient representatives. She could ask them to be involved, as they would be familiar with this role and could perhaps encourage and mentor other ex-patients who want to participate but lack, or have less confidence in having, the necessary skills. The problem with this approach is that it assumes that those issuing the invitations know the best people to ask, and it effectively excludes other people from participating. Sarah also wants to guard against the same people always being used, or being seen to be used, to represent patients (Cotterell et al. 2010, Rose et al. 2010). Seeking advice from others on who might be willing to work with them carries similar pros and cons. Nonetheless, Sarah thinks that it could be useful to contact the ex-ICU patients who are already involved in NHS trust matters, to see if they can recommend anyone who might be interested.

The third option, and the one Sarah's team tend to favour, is to ask for volunteers. Seeking volunteers makes it likely that those who offer to participate will be interested in working with the ICU team to develop services, and that all those within the group who are invited have an equal chance to participate. A disadvantage is that those who lack the confidence to put themselves forward are likely to be missed. In addition, those who were either very satisfied or very dissatisfied with their ICU experience are most likely to volunteer, with few people having middle-of-the-road opinions coming forward. Nonetheless, Sarah and her team think that asking for volunteers is more in keeping with the person-centred ethos of practice development than them deciding who to ask. It places the power to volunteer or not with ex-patients, not professionals, and means that everyone is equally entitled to become a part of the process of developing practice.

The practicalities of seeking volunteers is, however, a consideration for Sarah's team. After some thought, they decided to write to all the people who have been patients on the ICU over the past year and who have now been discharged from hospital, so that, as far as possible, each person has an equal opportunity to volunteer. This presents some practical challenges, such as people having relocated and not receiving the invitation. It also means that Sarah's team need to secure the resources and time to go through the processes required to access ex-patient names, identify their destinations after leaving hospital, and write to them.

Although volunteering is how Sarah and her team hope to achieve representation from ex-patients, they think that they may end up using a combination of volunteers and recommendations. Seeking volunteers will be their initial approach, but if not enough people come forward, those who do volunteer may be able to suggest or approach others to join the group. If they get too many volunteers, Sarah and her team plan to hold an event where those who have volunteered can hear more about what involvement will mean and then decide if they still wish to be part of the process. This will require time and physical resources such as a room and refreshments. However, the team feel that this approach will be the most congruent with the mutual respect and shared decision making they aim for, rather than them deciding who should be selected from all those who express an interest. It will also be consistent with the ethos of ex-patients being involved in the process of developing practice from the start, and throughout.

Practice pointer 5.7

Recruiting patient representatives can be achieved by:

- asking for volunteers
- approaching particular individuals
- seeking recommendations from others.

Recruitment strategies should include what to do if no one is interested in participating, and what to do if too many people volunteer.

Sarah and her team have considered whether to include the relatives of ICU patients in the process of developing practice. Person-centredness sees a person's social and societal position as an important part of who they are (Macleod and McPherson 2007). Families and significant others can also help practitioners to know the person they are caring for, their history and anticipated narrative, as well as their priorities, beliefs and values (Peek et al. 2007, Edvardsson et al. 2010, Thornton 2011). This may be especially relevant where a person has altered communication abilities and cannot tell their own story (Peek et al. 2007, McGilton et al. 2012). However, including families is always complicated by the need to ascertain who the person concerned would want to influence other people's perceptions of them, and the accuracy of those perceptions. The ICU team have, in the first instance, decided that they primarily want to understand the ICU experience from the patient's perspective. Thus, the initial invitation will be to ex-patients. They may involve families at a later stage, but this will depend on ex-patients' views, which seems to Sarah's team to be congruent with the ethos of ex-patients being involved in every decision that is made about how practice is developed.

Activity 5.4

If you were planning to involve patients in developing practice, who would you involve and how would you achieve this?

Involve from the start and throughout

Sarah and her team are committed to involving ex-patients throughout the process of developing practice. Although the idea to develop person-centred care began with them, they want to work with ex-patients at as early a stage as possible, so as to achieve real inclusion and equality of influence. As Chapter 4 discussed, practice development methodology focuses on developing depth of thinking, understanding of individuals and the achievement of mutual trust and respect. Sarah considers that the closer all participants are to beginning this process together, the more likely they are to achieve it.

Ex-patients being involved at as early a stage as possible will also mean that the whole process is more likely to be focused on what really matters to them, rather than on what practitioners assume is important (Braye and Preston-Shoot 2005, Diaz del Campo et al. 2011, Armstrong et al. 2013). In addition, ex-patients being a part of the whole process of developing practice will mean that as ideas develop, there will be an ongoing check of whether they match everyone's perspective of the initial vision (Braye and Preston-Shoot 2005).

However, although they want to involve ex-patients from the outset, Sarah's team have to consider what role they initially expect ex-patients to fulfil in the process of developing practice, so that they can be clear about this on the invitation to volunteer.

Defining roles and approaches

There are no hard-and-fast rules as to what roles patient representatives should play in developing practice, as these should be tailored to the nature of the proposed developments and the rationale for inviting patients to participate (Armstrong et al. 2013). Sarah's team do not have any concrete ideas about what particular roles people should adopt in the process of developing practice, and prefer the idea of enabling both staff and ex-patients who volunteer to develop particular responsibilities or interests that appeal to them (Armstrong et al. 2013). However, they need to be able to provide those who they invite to volunteer with a broad description of what the group will be expected to engage in, so that people can decide whether this is something they want to be a part of (Cotterell et al. 2010).

The team plans to include in the invitation letter how participants will be expected contribute to the development of practice. This will focus on people being prepared to share their experiences, explore with professionals how person-centred care might be developed and sustained, and be part of a group whose key principles will be mutual respect, dialogue and shared decision making. The letter will also state that no specific developments are currently planned, because the intention is for the people who participate to be involved in a process of determining how care can be improved. This will clarify what is expected of participants and the intention of the group (Cotterell et al. 2010).

Sarah's team think that a starting point of a partnership approach to developing practice will be for all concerned to agree some ground rules. These are likely to include the principles of equality and respect, and how they will jointly ensure a safe space and opportunities for negotiating and reaching decisions (Beresford 2010, TwoCan Associates 2011). They think that the first meeting will probably need to focus on this, and plan to indicate in the invitation letter that this is what participants should expect. So that people know what they are committing to practically, the letter will give the anticipated venue, duration and frequency of meetings.

Having decided what participants' roles will be, Sarah's team need to consider whether people will need any preparation for, or support in, fulfilling these roles.

Practice pointer 5.8

Those who participate in practice development initiatives should have information on:

* what they will be involved in
* the role they will be expected to play
* the level of commitment required.

Activity 5.5

What roles do you think patients could fulfil if they were involved in developing practice in your team?

Role preparation

Those involved in practice development activities, including staff and patients, may need preparation for and support in developing their roles in this process (Armstrong et al. 2013). Although equality of power and status between all participants is something Sarah is committed to, those participating might not all see this as a given, or be used to working in this way (Rise et al. 2013). Preparing people for, and developing their skills in achieving and sustaining, respectful relationships that facilitate partnership in decision making is something all concerned may require assistance and facilitation with (McCormack et al. 2007, Beresford 2010, TwoCan Associates 2011).

Critical social theory and critical realism, which inform practice development methodology, indicate the need to appreciate not just what the current status of an organization or system is, but how its history has contributed to this. In terms of achieving partnership with patients in developing practice, this includes how historical views of patients, by themselves and others, contribute to perspectives on their involvement in healthcare processes (Beresford 2010). Although her team's stated intention is to achieve genuine engagement with ex-patients, on an equal footing, Sarah is aware that some individuals may be influenced by patients' historical position as unequal partners in healthcare. Having been ICU patients may add to any inequality of status that ex-patients feel exists between themselves and professionals, and inhibit them from expressing their views. Equally, those whose ICU experience was less than satisfactory may find it difficult to achieve mutual respect and listen to healthcare professionals' views. At the same time, although the staff on the ICU generally subscribe to the concept of person-centredness, Sarah is unsure whether they are all committed to, or aware of, the reality and processes of achieving equal power, respect and shared decision making. A few casual comments she has heard on the unit suggest that this may not always be the case.

Evans et al. (2013) suggest that achieving effective patient involvement is often more challenging and takes more time than professionals initially anticipate. Sarah is committed to this ethos, but is not sure of her ability to facilitate and maintain it in others. She is therefore looking into a facilitator working with the group, not only to develop everyone's skills and confidence in critical reflection, but also to enable them to work together meaningfully. She needs to explore who might fulfil this role and how to procure funding for a facilitator's time.

Practice pointer 5.9

Staff and patients may need preparation for, and support in, the process of beginning to work together effectively to develop person-centred care.

Activity 5.6

What might you find challenging about patients being involved in the practice development process?

Valuing participation

Sarah thinks that a key part of demonstrating to ex-patients that their participation is valued will be that they are seen as equal partners, whose views and experiences are genuinely listened to and acted on. Another, more practical issue will be providing ex-patients with remuneration for any expenses incurred in participating, such as car parking fees (Evans et al. 2013). Evans et al. (2013) found that the non-financial outcomes of being involved in developing services are generally much more important to service users than financial ones. However, Sarah feels that payment to ex-patients for the expenses they incur is a reasonable expectation, and a resource she needs to secure. This is something she plans to clarify in the invitation letter, so that what will and will not be provided is clear and transparent from the outset.

Sarah thinks that what will really convince ex-patients that their participation is valued will be seeing that their input is acted on (Beresford 2010, Rose et al. 2010). She is also aware that real-world constraints mean that people's views or ideas may not always be able to be acted on, or not acted on immediately. She thinks that it is important to be clear from the outset that she cannot promise that everything will always be acted on as planned, and that change may be slower than people would like (TwoCan Associates 2011). What she thinks she can reasonably commit to is good communication, so that all group members know what is being done, what is not being done and why this is so. By working as a team, in which dialogue and mutual respect are key, she intends progress to be shared openly throughout the process of developing practice, including times where progress is delayed. This will mean that all participants know how their input is being used, and where it appears not to be influential, why this is (TwoCan Associates 2011). By striving to achieve equality of power, she also hopes that anyone, including ex-patients, will be able to challenge apparent delays in developments.

Practice pointer 5.10

When patients are involved in developing practice, there should be evidence that their views are listened to and acted on.

Summary

Sarah and her team have decided that it is in keeping with the person-centred focus of practice development methodology to involve ex-ICU patients at every stage of the practice development process. They aim to work in partnership with ex-patients so that meaningful dialogue can take place regarding what should and can be done to develop person-centred practice.

The key issues they think need to be considered in involving ex-patients in developing practice are:

- their rationale for involving ex-patients
- who they will involve

- how these people will be recruited
- what information potential participants will receive
- what preparation people will need for working together
- what resources will be needed to enable this to happen
- how they will ensure that ex-patients can see that their contributions are valued.

Having explored how ex-patients can meaningfully be involved in developing practice, Sarah is considering what information should influence developments. A key part of this is determining how the experiences and perceptions of ex-patients and practitioners can be used alongside other forms of evidence.

Case scenario

Kasia works as a children's community nurse specializing in supporting children who have complex health needs. She and her team have been considering how they can develop the support they provide so that it is more person centred, and Kasia is now exploring how they can involve the children and families who receive services in these developments. As well as this being a logical part of developing person-centred care, it seems to Kaisa to be an important part of empowering families. This has led her to consider why they might currently feel disempowered.

What might contribute to the children and families who Kaisa works with feeling disempowered?

The children Kaisa works with are likely to lack power because they are children and dependent on others for most of their day-to-day needs and care. In addition, because of their age and developmental level, they may find it difficult to make adults understand what they want to say. If their way of communicating is such that there are a limited number of people who are able to interact with them, they may be further disempowered. Children who have complex health needs are likely to be more dependent on others than their peers, which may further reduce their ability to control situations, and make them less inclined to challenge their carers. They may also have less social opportunities than other children, and therefore fewer chances to share their needs and preferences, and a smaller number of people with whom they can discuss these.

The parents Kaisa works with may feel disempowered because they have a heavy and continuous workload and many battles to fight, which leaves them little energy. They may be dependent on carers and thus feel disinclined to challenge them, and overwhelmed by health and social care processes that may seem to leave them few choices and limited control. Parents may also feel disempowered by not knowing exactly how systems work and why things happen as they do or decisions made as they are.

Thinking about the things that might disempower the families she works with has led Kaisa to consider what her aim in inviting families to participate in the process of developing practice is, whether it is primarily to empower them, or something else.

What would Kaisa's intention be in involving families in the practice development initiative? What term would she use to describe this?

Kaisa's main intention in involving families in developing practice is for them to contribute by sharing their experiences of care provision, how encounters make them feel and affect their lives, and their perceptions of events. However, despite this being clearly focused on them and their experiences, she also wants practitioners to be able to share their experiences, and how they perceive things, with families. Her goal is for this sharing to enable them to jointly explore developments that are focused on enhancing care as perceived by families, but which are also achievable for her team. She thinks that as well as developing practice, a better understanding of one another's perspectives may make working together easier for families and practitioners. Kaisa hopes that an effect of families working with staff on developing practice will be that they feel more empowered, but this is not the primary aim.

Kaisa wants to use the term 'partnership' to describe how she aims for her team to work with families, because she considers that this is what the approach she favours sets out to achieve.

Having decided why she wants to invite families to be involved, Kaisa is considering what the advantages and challenges of involving them in developing practice will be.

What will be the advantages and challenges in involving families in Kaisa's practice development initiative?

Involving families in developing practice may be beneficial because practitioners will be able to hear how parents and children perceive the care they are provided with, what is good about this and what would improve it. In addition, families may benefit from being able to hear how staff perceive things and what their experiences are. Staff and families meeting and engaging in dialogue about their perceptions and experiences may also mean that they have the chance get to know one another better as people. Kaisa thinks that this could enable practice to develop in a mutually beneficial way, with the individuals concerned better placed to understand one another.

Kaisa hopes that developing practice in partnership with families will help to keep the focus on developments that are important to them. When new challenges and competing priorities come along, families will be well placed to remind practitioners of what still matters to them.

Despite the benefits of seeking to work in partnership with families to develop practice, Kaisa can identify challenges to achieving this. These include:

- developing processes and approaches that mean that equality of power and mutual respect are achieved
- finding times and locations for meetings that are acceptable to families
- determining who should be involved and how they should be recruited
- the financial aspects of integrating families into the practice development process.

A further challenge will be to ensure that involvement is meaningful, not tokenistic, and that the benefits of working in partnership with families will be evident to them, but also to service providers.

How will Kaisa decide who to involve, and how will she achieve this?

Kaisa thinks that including parents and children in the practice development process is important, but in line with the person-centred nature of the intended developments, she will be guided on this by parents' and children's views. She wants to involve those who currently use services, so that the issues discussed are contemporary, and to include families whose care needs range from 24-hour care to shorter slots of care, as the issues may be different for each group.

Kaisa favours initially asking for volunteers. There are families she could approach, some of whom are already involved in patient engagement activities. However, she wants anyone to be able to participate, and does not want those who are already doing things to feel coerced to do more. She recognizes a possible difficulty in children being able to become involved, as both they and those with parental responsibility for them will need to agree to this. There may also be benefits in having separate discussion opportunities for children and parents. Equally, though, it could be useful, or practically necessary, to have one group that all interested parties attend. Kaisa thinks that the best thing will be to discuss with those who express an interest in participating how they think this should be managed, and what would be practical, as well as desirable, for most people.

What roles does Kaisa think families could fulfil in developing practice?

Kaisa thinks that the main role families will fulfil will be to share their experiences, perceptions, insights and what matters to them. They will, however, also need to be prepared to engage in mutually respectful discussions with professionals about differing perceptions, with the aim of developing practice.

In terms of commitment, families will need to be able to participate in discussions. Kaisa is considering whether alternatives to face-to-face contact, such as Skype, will be beneficial if parents or children find physical attendance difficult. If children who do not communicate verbally wish to participate, how their usual means of communication can be incorporated into discussions will need to be established.

Having considered some of the practicalities of integrating families into the process of developing practice, Kaisa has begun to think about what challenges this might present for her team.

What Kaisa's team might find challenging about family involvement in the practice development process

While Kaisa's team are, in theory, committed to working in partnership with families, the reality of it may prove challenging. Achieving the desired mutual respect may be difficult, and while hearing families' perspectives and experiences is, in theory, desirable, it may create feelings of insecurity or threat for individuals and the team as a whole. An additional challenge is that families will be able to hold practitioners to account for attempting to work in a more person-centred way on a day-to-day basis. Despite its desirability, this could be intimidating for staff.

Practitioners may be concerned that discussing incidents or viewpoints will upset or worry families, and be unsure of what to do if individuals want to discuss issues that involve families who are not there. The ground rules of discussions, including those of confidentiality and what can and cannot be shared, will therefore need to be clear. For this reason, as well as to facilitate reflective processes, Kaisa wants to secure the services of an external facilitator to work with the team on the process of developing a real partnership with families in developing practice

Additional resources

www.invo.org.uk
INVOLVE, a national advisory group that supports greater public involvement in NHS, public health and social care research.

www.kingsfund.org.uk/projects/gp-inquiry/patient-engagement-involvement
Page of the King's Fund website that focuses on encouraging patient involvement in the design, planning and delivery of health services.

www.rcn.org.uk/development/practice/principles/principle_d
Page of the Royal College of Nursing website that discusses Principle D, involving patients in healthcare.

6 What Informs Practice Development?

Chapter overview

- The focus of practice development methodology is on knowing people, and developing practice based on this knowledge. The evidence that it uses centres on understanding the beliefs, values, perceptions and priorities of patients, their relatives and practitioners, and the effect that people's social and cultural situations have on them.
- Practice development methodology also uses knowledge gained from research, audit, evaluation, expert opinion, case reports and clinical guidelines.
- In order to base developments in practice on good evidence, the right type and quality of evidence should be used for the right thing, and evidence from across sources collated, to give as full and in depth an understanding as possible to decision making.

Hannah works as a practice nurse in a large city centre practice. The practice has become concerned about the number of their patients who present at the accident and emergency (A&E) department when they could have used the practice's services. Hannah has been considering how to develop the practice's provision so that it centres on the needs of those using the service, thus making the practice a more attractive option. As a result, she has developed a proposal for practice nurses to offer a walk-in triage service for people who do not have appointments. This would involve a practice nurse deciding whether the person could be given advice and input by them, needed to see a GP, or required hospital care.

Hannah has used the principles of practice development methodology to inform her approach to gathering and collating the information that has resulted in this proposal, and is now preparing to explain her ideas and how they have been developed. The starting point of her proposal arose from practice-based knowledge gleaned from patients, colleagues and her own experiences and reflections.

Personal and practice-based knowledge

Practice development methodology focuses on developing practice in a way that meets the needs of the people who receive care, as perceived by them. It therefore sees the knowledge, understanding, beliefs, values, perceptions and priorities of these people as crucial forms of evidence (McCormack et al. 2009). Hannah considered the knowledge, experiences, understanding, beliefs, values, perceptions and priorities of those who chose to visit A&E rather than the practice as critical to understanding the best way to develop services. She thought this was the information that would really give her an idea of what might or might not encourage people to use and be satisfied with the practice's services. Without this knowledge, the practice could easily spend time and effort developing a service that, however well intentioned and planned, did not address the needs of those using the service and therefore did not reduce inappropriate A&E attendances.

As Chapter 5 discussed, involving patients at the earliest possible stage of developing practice is valuable because it enables developments to be focused on what matters to them. Thus, Hannah began her enquiries about what made people use A&E instead of the practice by convening a discussion group with patients. She invited people whose records indicated they had attended A&E within the last six months, when they could perhaps have used the practice's services, to an informal group meeting to share their views and experiences. Fifteen people attended, which surprised Hannah, as she had expected considerably less. She used this opportunity to ask if anyone would like to be involved in developing an innovation aimed at improving what the practice could offer. Five people expressed an interest.

Activity 6.1

How could you access information about what patients and their relatives think is good about the care your team provides, and what could be improved?

Practice pointer 6.1

Practice development methodology sees the knowledge, understanding, beliefs, values, perceptions and priorities of the people who receive care as important elements of the evidence that should inform practice.

Centring developments in practice on the perceptions of those who are on the receiving end of care is the cornerstone of practice development methodology. However, as Chapter 2 identified, practice development methodology sees people's perceptions and actions as being influenced by a complex mix of group as well as individual beliefs, values, norms, and the social and historical context in which events happen (Bergin et al. 2008, Freeman and Vasconcelos 2010, Oliver 2012, Parlour and McCormack 2012). Hannah therefore sought to explore not just what symptoms or apparent circumstances led people to decide to use A&E rather than the practice, but why this was and what influenced their decisions. One person explained that they went to A&E because they had been spoken to abruptly and made to feel like a time waster when they tried to make an emergency appointment at the practice. They also commented that several of their friends had reported similar experiences. Regardless of whether or not the staff who had spoken to this person had intended to be, or had been, abrupt, this was the individual's perception. Her interpretation of events might also have been influenced by what others in her social group had reported to her, but they were still her perceptions. These perceptions and experiences would need to be addressed in any developments in practice, so that she and other people felt welcome at any new service that was offered. Another person said that it was accepted wisdom among her work colleagues that it was better to use A&E than the practice for anything urgent, as appointments with GPs were difficult to organize. She therefore only visited the practice for routine screening or prescriptions and did not attempt to make appointments for other matters. This indicated to Hannah that as well as developing a particular service, the practice would need to provide clear, accessible, consistent information about it so that patients knew of its existence and purpose. Otherwise, what the practice had historically offered, and what people's peers and colleagues told them, would continue to direct where they sought healthcare.

Activity 6.2

What are your views on the care provided in your workplace?

Hannah considered this form of evidence critical, because unless developments in practice were based on what those who might use any new service perceived and saw as important, they would still bypass the practice and attend A&E. However, as Chapters 2 and 3 identified, person-centred practice development methodology also recognizes practitioners as key people in developments in practice (McCormack and McCance 2006, Manley and McCormack 2008). Hannah's own experiences, views, beliefs, values, priorities and perceptions and those of the rest of the practice team were also important sources of information regarding why things were as they were now, and whether they could be altered (McCormack 2008). This included not just people's experiences while working in this practice, but their previous experiences, and how the views of each individual within the group influenced the perceptions of the others.

Hannah reflected on her experiences in a previous post in an A&E department: how she had perceived people who attended inappropriately, why they said they attended, and sometimes the distinction between why they said they attended and their real reason for attendance. She also considered her current work, how she felt about and responded to people who attended for various types of appointments, and what might encourage or discourage patients from using the practice's services. As well as this, she thought about how other people in the practice team seemed to perceive certain types of attendance and the way in which patients were spoken to or given advice. In addition, Hannah pondered how individual people's perceptions might influence the views of the team as a whole. She then asked her colleagues, including the other practice nurses, GPs and the reception staff, their views on these issues, so as to build as complete as possible a picture of what mattered to the people involved in providing the practice's services.

Activity 6.3

How could you seek your colleagues' views on what is good, what works well and what could be improved in your workplace?

Practice pointer 6.2

The experiences, views, beliefs, values, priorities and perceptions of practitioners are important sources of knowledge in person-centred practice development.

After Hannah had gathered the perspectives of staff and patients, she looked for a way to present the key issues and clarify how all this evidence fitted together. As Chapter 2 outlined, critical social theory identifies three types of knowledge: technical interest, practical interest and emancipatory interest (Habermas 1971). Although critical social theory is only one element of the underpinnings of practice development methodology, Hannah found these three types of interest or knowledge a useful way to organize and present this aspect of her evidence.

Habermas's (1971) first type of knowledge concerns technical knowledge and skills. In Hannah's case, this included:

- patients' knowledge about the available services and their purpose
- their skills in managing their own conditions
- the skills and knowledge practitioners thought they had or could offer
- the knowledge and skills they felt they would need to develop if alternative services were offered.

This was useful to Hannah in identifying what people thought was available, what they felt they could or could not currently do and why, and what additional knowledge, skills or resources might be needed in order for practice to develop.

Habermas's (1971) second type of knowledge is practical knowledge, which concerns how others see their world. This sort of information goes beyond what should, technically, work well, to what things mean to people and how this will affect what they are prepared to do or engage with. A significant proportion of the information that Hannah had collected about staff and patients' perceptions comprised this type of knowledge. She saw this as crucial in terms of determining whether any developments in what the practice could offer would be likely to be acceptable and seen as useful by patients, and acceptable for and therefore adopted by staff. It also enabled the reasons behind these perceptions to be understood, so that they could be addressed if necessary.

Habermas's (1971) third type of knowledge, emancipatory interest, addresses understanding oneself and how the world in which one functions is influenced by social conditions. It relates to knowledge about the things within individuals, but also in the world in which they live and work, which influences their perception of themselves, their present and past experiences, and their level of empowerment (Bevan et al. 2012). Hannah's evidence in this case included:

- awareness of how her own experiences, assumptions, values and priorities influenced how she perceived people who attended A&E when they could have used the practice's services
- how she felt about her work and workplace
- how she perceived her colleagues and their responses to patients
- what her motivations for wanting to develop practice were.

Emancipatory knowledge also addresses issues of power. As Chapters 2 and 3 identified, the power that individuals and groups hold in particular situations is seen as important in critical realism and critical social theory (Freeman and Vasconcelos 2010, Bevan et al. 2012, Lapum et al. 2012). Hannah thought that the power equations that existed, or were felt to exist, between patients and staff were therefore important. However, power issues between staff within the practice (including power between groups of staff and individual staff) and between the practice and the wider social and political environment in terms of regulations and resources were equally important considerations.

Box 6.1 provides a summary of how Hannah grouped the information she had gained into these three forms of knowledge. She thought that these matched the ethos of practice development methodology. However, she had also accessed other forms of evidence, such as research and expert opinion, and wanted to present these alongside her practice-based observations, enquiries and reflections. As she considered how to present the information she had gathered, she came across the concept of hierarchies of evidence, but her way of viewing the evidence she had collected did not seem to fit particularly well with these.

Box 6.1 How Hannah used Habermas's (1971) types of knowledge to inform developments in practice

Technical knowledge and skills

Patients' knowledge about available services and their purpose

Patient's skills in managing their own conditions

Practitioners' existing skills and knowledge

Practitioners' perceived skills and knowledge deficits for new services

Any threat practitioners might perceive from new services developing

Practical knowledge

Practitioners' perceptions of the services currently provided

Patients' perceptions of the services currently provided

What works for practitioners

Why practitioners see these things as working well

What works for patients

Why patients see these things as working well

What does not work well for practitioners

Why practitioners do not see these things as working well

What does not work for patients

Why patients do not see these things as working well

What patients would see as good about particular developments

What patients would see as problematic about particular developments

What practitioners would see as good about particular developments

What practitioners would see as problematic about particular developments

Emancipatory knowledge

Hannah's experiences

Hannah's thoughts, beliefs and assumptions about the services currently provided, her colleagues and patients

Hannah's values

Hannah's priorities

The power equations that practitioners perceive exist

The power equations that patients perceive exist

Practitioners' views on regulations, funding and resources

Hierarchies of evidence

Hierarchies of evidence are essentially guidance on the principle values of different types of evidence, and are primarily designed for use in developing such things as guidelines and protocols. Because their intention is to suggest the best action to take in most instances of a particular situation, they work on the premise that the best form of evidence is that which is most generalizable (NICE 2005). As a result, meta-analyses, randomized controlled trials and other forms of quantitative research are usually at the top of hierarchies of evidence. This makes sense when the intention is to comment on the best form of generalizable evidence, but is less helpful for situations where this is not the aim.

Using one hierarchy to determine the quality of all evidence is problematic because the quality of evidence is, in part, dependent on what it is being used for and in what context (Cruickshank 2012). The sole use of evidence such as randomized controlled trials to inform practice presumes that an intervention that produced a particular set of outcomes will produce those outcomes in every situation. This does not take into account, as, for instance, critical realism does, the many factors in a particular situation that might interact to make something work or not (Cruickshank 2012, Oliver 2012). Hannah had found a piece of quantitative research that seemed useful for informing developments in her workplace's practice. However, she felt that its application should be guided by the information she had gathered about her particular practice situation. Otherwise, even good quality research might not provide solutions that worked effectively in her practice's circumstances. In addition, the principle of practice development methodology is that it begins with and focuses around what matters to the individual people in the situation in question, rather than beginning with the external evidence that exists.

Practice pointer 6.3

Hierarchies of evidence:

- give guidance on the principle value of different types of evidence
- are primarily designed to show what type of evidence is the most safely generalizable
- usually place highly generalizable research at the top of the hierarchy
- are not always helpful when generalizability is not the aim.

The evidence that informs practice development activities can, and should, draw on published information about what has been shown to work and what has not worked. However, no evidence, however compelling or brilliant, should be seen in isolation. The critical realist perspective that informs practice development methodology sees perceptions of reality as largely socially constructed. As such, practice development should combine evidence from sources such as research with knowledge from a range of other, more personal and contextual sources to determine what might work best in a particular situation (Harwood and Clark 2012, Oliver 2012). Consequently, the value of each type of evidence in developing practice is not determined by a preordained hierarchy, but its value in a given situation and in conjunction with other sources of information.

Practice development methodology aims to integrate the development of evidence from practice and the use of evidence in practice (McCormack et al. 2013). Using empirical evidence and other sources of written information can, therefore, help practice developers to question why things are done as they are, challenge their assumptions, and give them ideas about what could be done differently (Aleem et al. 2009, Hahn 2009, Sanders et al. 2013). Knowing the worth of any type of evidence and how suitable it is likely to be to inform the development in question is useful.

Practice pointer 6.4

In practice development:

• no evidence should be seen in isolation
• evidence from a variety of sources should be used
• evidence from practice should be integrated with the use of evidence in practice.

Research

Research has been defined as a rigorous and systematic process of gathering and analysing information, resulting in new knowledge being generated (Burton 2004, Hewitt-Taylor 2011). However, what constitutes a rigorous and systematic approach depends on what information is being sought and for what purpose. A distinction is usually made between qualitative and quantitative research: both are research, but their intention and thus the criteria for judging their quality are very different. Qualitative research (also referred to as 'naturalistic' or 'interpretivist' research) aims to achieve in-depth exploration of human experiences. Its intention is generally to enhance understanding of individual and subjective things like feelings, values or beliefs. As such, it acknowledges that the 'truth' may be subjective and interpreted differently by different people or in different circumstances (LoBiondo-Wood and Haber 2005). To gain the type of understanding that qualitative research aspires to, the researcher seeks to build up an in-depth picture of what is being studied and the context of the study. This should enable those reading the research report to decide how its findings might apply to their situation. Qualitative research accepts subjectivity, does not aim to find an answer that can be confidently applied to everyone in a given population, and does not, therefore, seek generalizability (Kearney 2005, LoBiondo-Wood and Haber 2005, Goodman 2008). The key issues in the quality of qualitative research are whether enough depth of enquiry and detailed understanding of individual situations and experiences has been achieved.

Hannah found a qualitative study about the experiences of people who chose to use A&E in situations where they could have used their practice. The study explored issues such as:

- how people made these decisions
- what they expected in healthcare provision
- what they valued in services
- how they viewed their health.

The research showed the complexity of people's decision-making processes, but did not aim to develop a generalizable intervention, which would work in every situation. It gave Hannah useful additional insights to add to her own observations and conversations with colleagues to help her understand what might influence people's decisions, and what mattered to them in service provision. The contextual descriptions of the study location and participants seemed to match hers quite well. She therefore thought that, although the study was not intended to be generalizable to all practice situations, it did have some resonance with and transferability to hers.

Quantitative research, sometimes also referred to as 'positivist research', quantifies things, so, unlike qualitative enquiry, which mainly uses words to describe experiences, it uses numbers. The belief underpinning quantitative research is that truth is objective, not dependent on context or interpretation, and that by using numbers, one can show whether or not something works (McGrath and Johnson 2003, Lee 2006). It aims to use statistical analysis to predict how likely it is that its findings should apply, equally, to most people within a certain population or group, referred to as 'generalizability' (Lee 2006). The design of a quantitative study should therefore aim to make its findings as generalizable as possible, within a given population. These beliefs contrast with the underpinning principles of qualitative research; thus the two cannot be judged using the same criteria.

Among the evidence she had collected, Hannah had a quantitative study of the outcomes of a practice introducing a practice nurse triaging system. This detailed:

- what the intervention was
- how many patients were seen

- the outcomes of the triaging process
- the number of patients inappropriately attending A&E in the three months following the introduction of the new system
- a comparison with the picture in the preceding three months.

This provided quantifiable evidence of the possible benefits of this type of service, as the study showed that the number of inappropriate A&E attendances reduced after the introduction of the triaging service. It also gave the number of triaged patients who needed to be seen by a GP, which would be useful for Hannah in service planning. The study's statistical analysis showed that the results were significant, which enabled Hannah to assume that these findings could, with some confidence, be applied to her workplace.

There is also an increasing interest in what is referred to as 'mixed methods' research (Bryman 2006, Halcomb et al. 2009). This means that a study uses a combination of qualitative and quantitative approaches, and is useful when what needs to be investigated requires both quantification and consideration of qualitative aspects of a subject in order for it to be understood (Johnson and Onwuegbuzie 2004, Halcomb et al. 2009). Mixed methods research differs from two separate studies that use different methodologies because it is one study that gathers data using different perspectives on a subject to provide an overall picture. This approach is often useful for informing developments in practice as it can combine statistical information with an exploration of the personal and contextual factors that may affect the acceptability or success of a particular way of working. Hannah had one mixed methods study in the evidence she had collated, which explored the implementation of a system of practice nurses offering a walk-in service to patients who did not have appointments. It quantified how many patients attended, the length of appointments, the outcomes of their consultations, and the number who then went on to have GP appointments or attend A&E. In addition, it used qualitative methods of data collection and analysis to explore the practice nurses' views of this service, so as to determine whether the system was acceptable to them. This gave a useful overall picture of how far this type of service might improve provision, but also what would need to be put in place to make it achievable and sustainable from staff perspectives.

Activity 6.4

What do you think qualitative and quantitative research could add to your knowledge about how your workplace could develop practice?

> **Practice pointer 6.5**
>
> • Research should be rigorous, systematic and use an appropriate approach for the subject in question.
> • Quantitative research is useful when the intention is to measure a phenomenon.
> • Qualitative research is useful when the intention is to study subjective, non-generalizable issues such as human experiences, feelings, values or beliefs.
> • Mixed methods research is useful when what is being investigated needs a combination of qualitative and quantitative approaches.

No methodological approach to research is inherently superior to another, what matters is whether it is right for what is being investigated and whether a systematic and rigorous process was used to conduct the enquiry. Exactly what should be checked to determine the quality of any study depends on the type of study in question. However, the type of questions it is useful to consider when evaluating research include:

• Was the type of research used appropriate for the issue being studied?
• Were the methods, that is, the ways the information was collected, congruent with this? For example, in qualitative research, were interviews conducted in enough depth? In quantitative research, were measurements appropriate and accurate?
• Were the ways of analysing the data appropriate? For example, were the right statistical tests used to analyse quantitative data?
• Was the whole process rigorous and systematic?

Box 6.2 shows some general principles that can be used to evaluate research. There are also various tools that can be used to evaluate the quality of particular types of research. One such set of tools are the Critical Appraisal Skills Programme (CASP) tools (www.caspinternational.org/?o=1012).

Box 6.2 General principles of evaluating research

What the study is about
Study title/hypothesis/question/statement of intent

Study background
Does the literature review/background appear unbiased and relevant to the study?

Study paradigm, design and methodology
Do the study paradigm, methodology and design fit the subject?
Are the paradigm, design and methodology congruent with each other?

Methods

Do these seem a reasonable approach to finding the information required?

Does the way the methods were used match the methodology/paradigm?

Does anything about the methods seem likely to produce misleading results?

Were any procedures or tools developed appropriately, for example piloted, discussed with experts?

Sample

Was the sample and the way it was selected appropriate?

Would the way in which the sample was selected have placed any limitations on the results?

Was the response rate high enough (if relevant)?

Ethical issues

Were the ethical issues involved in the study considered? This might include ethics review, informed consent, coercion to participate, potential harm, confidentiality and anonymity.

Data analysis

Was the right approach to data analysis used?

Were appropriate specific analysis procedures used? For example, which statistical tests were used and were these appropriate?

Reliability and validity/trustworthiness

Does it appear that the study was conducted systematically?

Was anything obvious missing?

Was there anything that might have meant that the results could be misleading or due to something other than what was being investigated?

For quantitative research

Were reliability, internal validity, in terms of construct validity, content validity and criterion validity (where appropriate), and external validity addressed?

Were all the data accounted for – no missing results?

For qualitative research

Are the steps the researcher took to ensure the 'truth' of their findings clear?

For mixed methods research

Were the data analysis processes appropriate for the type of data in question, and was there evidence of appropriate integration of findings?

Results/findings
Are these clearly related to the study title/hypothesis/question/statement of intent?
Are they consistent with the methodology, methods and sampling?
Are any other things that might have influenced the results accounted for?

Conclusions and recommendations
Do the conclusions and recommendations match the findings?
Are the conclusions presented with the appropriate degree of certainty, given the methodology, methods and findings?

Source: Adapted from Hewitt-Taylor 2011

Practice pointer 6.6

Research is only a good form of evidence if:

- it uses the right methodology and methods for what it is exploring
- it is systematically and rigorously conducted.

Hannah used the CASP tool for qualitative research to evaluate the qualitative study that she found. The quantitative study did not seem to fit a particular CASP tool, so she used the general principles of evaluating quantitative research instead. For the mixed methods study, she used the CASP tool to evaluate the qualitative element, the principles of evaluating quantitative research to evaluate the quantitative part, but also considered how the two aspects of the study were integrated and informed each other and how this affected the overall quality of the study.

Although an individual study can provide valuable information, it is also important is to look at the evidence from across studies, to see whether there are patterns, consistencies or inconsistencies that can be highlighted. One of the forms of evidence that can be valuable in this respect is a systematic review.

Systematic reviews

A systematic review is a systematic and rigorous review of the available evidence on a particular subject. Such reviews generally appear high up in hierarchies of evidence, because they should, if performed diligently, provide a composite picture of the evidence from across studies. Because they present the findings from across several studies, with a commentary on their quality and the strength of the overall evidence, they are often regarded as a higher form of evidence than a single piece of research.

The term 'systematic review', like the term 'research', covers a number of different techniques and approaches to cater for the synthesis of different types of research. These include meta-analysis, meta-synthesis, narrative synthesis and mixed methods synthesis:

1 *Meta-analysis* is a quantitative technique, which uses statistical methods to show how confidently a recommendation for using a particular approach can be made. It effectively summarizes quantitative data from two or more studies where the outcomes being measured and how they are being measured is identical (Crombie and Davies 2009, Deeks et al. 2011). It usually uses data from randomized controlled trials, although there is discussion about whether non-randomized data can also be used (Crombie and Davies 2009, Deeks et al. 2011). By combining data from across studies, meta-analysis effectively increases the sample size being considered and can therefore give a more precise estimate of the effect of an intervention than any of the individual studies included in the analysis can (Deeks et al. 2011). Meta-analyses are often placed at the top of hierarchies of evidence because they are, in principle, the most generalizable form of evidence. However, they are only the best form of evidence when used for something suitable for a meta-analysis and if that meta-analysis is well performed. Hannah had only found one quantitative and one mixed methods study about developing a nurse triage system in GP practices. It was therefore unsurprising she did not find any relevant meta-analyses, because the type of data required for these to be conducted was unlikely to exist.

2 *Meta-synthesis* is the umbrella term used for the process of synthesizing qualitative data. Meta-analysis is not a suitable approach for synthesizing qualitative data because it employs statistical procedures (Dixon-Woods et al. 2006). Several different techniques for achieving this exist, but the aim is to develop, enlarge or broaden understanding of the phenomenon under investigation rather than achieve greater clarity over the generalizability of the findings from across studies (Barnett-Page and Thomas 2009). Hannah did not find any qualitative systematic reviews, which was to be expected, given that she had only found one relevant qualitative study (related to why people used A&E rather than their practices) and one mixed methods study (about a practice developing a nurse triaging system).

3 *Narrative synthesis* encompasses a range of approaches to synthesizing the evidence from across research studies. Although it can use numerical methods, the focus is on the use of words and descriptions to explain and summarize the findings. However, while a range of processes can be used in narrative synthesis, each synthesis should be systematic and the reasons for the decisions made in it transparent (Rodgers et al. 2009, Deeks et al. 2011).

4 *Mixed methods synthesis* is used when a question requires the synthesis of both qualitative and quantitative research to answer it. Like narrative synthesis, it can use a variety of approaches in order to achieve this, but requires the processes used to be systematic and the decisions made to be clear and appropriate for the question being addressed (Sandelowski et al. 2012). Hannah had not found any narrative or mixed methods syntheses, which was as she expected, given that she had not found very much research on this subject.

Despite being regarded as a highly valuable form of evidence, a systematic review, like research, is only good if it is well conducted, and only useful insofar as it is applicable to a particular area of practice. The key issues to use to judge the quality of a systematic review have been suggested by CASP (2010).

In addition to research and systematic reviews, audit and evaluation can be useful sources of evidence for informing developments in practice and have many similarities to research in terms of process.

Practice pointer 6.7

A systematic review:

* provides a composite picture of evidence from across a range of studies
* is only good quality evidence if it is well conducted
* is only useful where it is applicable.

Activity 6.5

Visit a site that allows access to systematic reviews, such as the Joanna Briggs Institute (http://joannabriggs.org/index.html) or The Cochrane Library (www. thecochranelibrary.com/view/0/index.html). Do they have any reviews relevant to your practice? If not, why might this be? If so, of what value would these be to you in developing practice?

Audit and evaluation

Hannah had found two papers that were described as an audit and an evaluation of the services provided by practices. The evaluation paper turned out not to be relevant to her current practice development activities, but the audit was. However, having read them, she was not entirely sure how they differed from the papers described as research. Audit and evaluation have many similarities to research: they all gather and analyse information and should all follow systematic and rigorous processes (Wade 2005). The distinction between the three is often described (Wade 2005, NPSA/NRES 2009) as being that:

- *research* investigates what should be done
- *audit* investigates whether or not what should be done is being done
- *evaluation* examines how useful or effective something is, or what standard it achieves.

Research may involve trialling a new intervention, with a view to using it in the future if it is shown to work well. In contrast, audit and evaluation involve an intervention or interventions that are being used regardless of the audit or evaluation activity, although the outcomes of the audit or evaluation may influence their ongoing use (NPSA/NRES 2009). Audit and evaluation should be carried out as systematically and rigorously as research and, like research, should use processes appropriate for what they intend to investigate or achieve. Because of their similarities to research in terms of process and tools, the criteria used for evaluating research can often be applied to elements of evaluation and audit.

Hannah had found an audit of a service where patients could telephone the practice nurses between 9 and 11 each day, to gain advice on how to proceed with their needs. The audit aimed to identify how many calls were taken, the outcome of those calls, and the destination of the patients concerned, for example A&E, GP appointment, a visit to or further advice from the practice nurse. Although this was an audit of an existing service, not research, it seemed sensible to Hannah to base her appraisal of it on the principles of evaluating research. She thought that the quality issues would be similar in terms of the study being systematic and rigorous, albeit with some necessary differences in how the setting and sample were selected, and how approval to conduct the audit was obtained.

Practice pointer 6.8

- Research investigates what should be done.
- Audit investigates whether or not what should be done is being done.
- Evaluation examines how useful or effective something is, or what standard it achieves.

Hannah had also collected one paper described as 'action research', which seemed to her to be a hybrid of research and evaluation.

Action research

Action research involves practitioners looking at their own practice, instigating something that might improve or develop this, and then using research techniques to evaluate the effects of this development (Ferrance 2000, Parkin 2009). It is generally seen as congruent with practice development, insofar as practitioners identify an area for development, action is planned, followed by evaluation of and reflection on that action. Where necessary and appropriate, further refinement of the original plan, with ongoing evaluation and development, continues this process (Parkin 2009).

Action research has similarities to both research and evaluation: the techniques of research are used, but these are interlinked with a real-world innovation in practice being developed and evaluated, followed by further developments and evaluations (Parkin 2009). It is also strongly linked with the principles and processes of practice development methodology. A key element of action research is that it is participatory: it is research with rather than on the people concerned (Borg et al. 2012). As such, action research is carried out by practitioners, not on them, and may, where appropriate, include patients working in partnership with practitioners throughout the process. Similarly, as Chapter 5 identified, practitioners and patients should work together to develop person-centred practice. Borg et al. (2012) highlight the importance of reflection and reflexivity in action research, as those who are the researchers are also intimately involved with the subject of the research and the context in which it takes place. This again links with the reflection and reflexivity of practice development methodology described in Chapter 4.

The paper Hannah had found that was described as action research reported how nurses in a particular practice developed an evening drop-in service because they identified that people often attended A&E instead of their practice in the evenings. The team developing the new service included two patient representatives. The development was evaluated by numerically assessing numbers of attendees, but also by exploring the views of a group of patients who attended, the development team reflecting on their own experiences of the development and provision of the service, and seeking feedback from their colleagues through semi-structured interviews. Hannah thought that the paper described something very like a mix of evaluation and research processes, with a strong link to mixed methods research. However, she could also see how it was firmly embedded in practice, with anticipated ongoing cycles of development and evaluation as the initiative was refined and further developed. Having considered this report, Hannah realized that the innovation she was proposing had the potential to be a form of action research.

Hannah now had a collection of evidence that spanned her own, her colleagues' and patients' experiences, and various forms of enquiry such as research, audit and action research. She had also come across some other forms of evidence, including one guideline from another practice related to practice nurses triaging patients.

Practice pointer 6.9

Action research:

- arises from a practice-based issue
- involves instigating something that might improve or develop practice
- uses research techniques to evaluate that development
- is cyclical – initial evaluation is followed by further refinement, action and evaluation.

Clinical guidelines

Clinical guidelines are recommendations, based on the best available evidence, about what is considered to be the most appropriate treatment or care for the majority of people with a specific disease or condition, and what should be done in practice because of that evidence (NICE 2009). Like every other form of evidence, a guideline is only as good as the information in it and the way in which that information has been interpreted and presented. A clinical guideline that provides a high-quality systematic analysis of all the available evidence and presents this in a logical sequence accompanied by details of its practical application is likely to be very useful. However, a guideline that provides no more information than what should be done is less useful because the reader does not know the basis on which they should do this.

Guidelines are intended to provide information to direct what should be done in most instances of a given situation. Generalizable evidence is therefore usually considered the best form of evidence from which to develop them. However, all guidelines tend to come with the caveat that they should be interpreted and applied according to the specific needs and nuances of each individual or circumstance.

The guideline Hannah had found was for practice nurses carrying out a preliminary assessment of patients. It indicated what practice nurses should do in terms of assessment and referral pathways, but it did not state the quality of evidence it was drawn from or why these actions should be taken. This was almost inevitable, because the existing evidence was likely to be minimal, and the guideline seemed intended to be a quick reference guide for people to use in day-to-day situations, rather than a lengthy document. The guideline was therefore useful to help Hannah identify the practical considerations that would be necessary if her team adopted this kind of innovation, but the quality of its recommendations was difficult for her to evaluate.

Hannah also had one case report in the evidence she had collected.

Case reports

Case reports usually report a case or cases of a particular condition, disorder, disease or situation, detail what happened in that case, analyse this, and suggest and debate alternative explanations for it. However, they do not generally adopt such a systematic, detailed or rigorous process as research (Gopikrishna 2010). For this reason, they are, in principle, usually regarded as lower quality sources of information than systematic reviews, research, audit or evaluation. Nevertheless, like all forms of evidence, their value depends on their inherent quality, what they are being used for, and why. For example, a detailed and diligently considered case report could constitute better evidence than a poorly conducted, methodologically flawed piece of research. Hannah had found one case report of a person who had attended a practice where an advanced nurse practitioner saw him and was able to assess his needs, manage these herself, review him the next day, and avoid him attending A&E or needing a GP appointment. Because the report detailed exactly what had led the person to present at the practice and the way the advanced nurse practitioner had assessed and managed the situation, Hannah was able to think about aspects of that service she would want to replicate. Thus, while it was not generalizable, it was a useful addition to her body of evidence because it was a detailed, well-written report.

Expert opinion

Expert opinion is exactly what it says it is, the opinion of an expert or experts in a particular field of work. While this can be a valuable source of information, the basis for claims to expertise varies and thus the value of expert opinion is variable. Expert opinion is not usually considered to be as strong a form of evidence as research, because the views of experts may not be a result of the systematic approach to enquiry that is demanded in research (Gopikrishna 2010). Consensus expert opinion is generally seen as preferable to an individual's view, because it is less likely to be subjective. Often, case reports and expert opinion are combined, as an expert in the field will provide a case report, in which they use their expertise to analyse the key issues involved in that case. Hannah did not think that she had come across any of this type of written evidence, although the case report she had read was written by someone who seemed to be an expert in their field of practice, and thus probably spanned both types of evidence.

Practice pointer 6.10

Guidelines, case reports and expert opinion can all be useful forms of evidence. The key to their value is their quality and what they are being used for.

Activity 6.6

What might guidelines, case reports and expert opinion add to your knowledge about developing practice in your workplace?

Fitting all the evidence together

Although each piece of evidence Hannah had collected had its own value, she had to collate all the evidence from across these sources to develop an overall picture of what it seemed appropriate to do, and why. For Hannah, a key factor in her decisions was not just the quality of each piece of evidence, but its relevance to her situation, and to what the people she had spoken to said mattered to them (Regan 2011). Where she used research, guidelines and case reports, she noted their quality, but also their applicability to her situation, and how the different pieces of evidence corroborated or contradicted each other. She then linked this to the evidence she had gathered from her practice-based enquiry and observations. Her overall review of the evidence can be seen in Box 6.3.

Box 6.3 Evidence to support the development of a nurse-led, walk-in triage service for patients who do not have appointments

Evidence from practice

Practitioners (including self): Would prefer patients to use the practice rather than A&E, sometimes find it irritating when patients misuse emergency appointments, find that patients sometimes claim to be attending for a reason other than their presenting problem so as to secure an appointment, feel limited in what they can offer patients whose needs are neither urgent nor routine, can appreciate that patients want more flexibility in the timing of appointments but cannot offer this, are not certain what a nurse-led triage system would mean, nurses are not all confident that they could triage patients effectively but most are willing and feel able to learn these skills, GPs feel confident that nurses could learn these skills and are willing to assist in their development.

Patients: Would prefer to attend the practice rather than A&E as it is a more convenient location, may be seen as time wasters in A&E but at least they will be seen that day, GP appointments are tightly controlled whereas in A&E patients have more power to be seen when they consider it to be necessary, difficult to negotiate an appointment at the practice when they find it hard to explain symptoms, sometimes feel that practice staff regard them as using emergency appointments inappropriately but cannot get other appointments in a timely manner, may have to 'talk symptoms up' to get seen, unsure what an 'emergency' is in the practice's terms, think that it is too difficult to arrange GP appointments except for very routine matters, attend A&E if unsure how to manage their condition but unable to get a prompt appointment at the practice, the time slots for appointments at the practice do not fit their needs.

Conclusions: Practitioners and patients would prefer the practice rather than A&E to be used. There is a gap in provision for patients who need help with assessing their needs or whose needs/perceived needs do not neatly match a standard GP appointment or A&E attendance. A&E is currently seen as providing a more flexible service, particularly for needs people find hard to categorize. Practitioners are generally willing to explore new ways of working in order to overcome this problem.

Qualitative research

People who chose to use A&E rather than their practices generally saw A&E as a valid alternative if accessing an appointment with a GP was difficult: this included difficulty in finding convenient time slots for appointments, not wanting to miss work for important but non-life-threatening illnesses, and accessing an appointment in a timely fashion. People would have preferred to see their GP as they were generally located more conveniently, would know them, and had their records. Some people viewed their health as a peripheral part of their lives and delayed seeing a GP until it was urgent and their symptoms were unbearable. Conversely, some people felt that the response of practices was not urgent or rapid enough and therefore attended A&E with what were ultimately considered to be minor symptoms.

The reasons people went to A&E instead of using their practice's services ranged from expecting prompt attention and going to A&E when this was not forthcoming to expecting there to be no GP appointments available and opting to go directly to A&E without enquiring about what their practice could offer.

Conclusions: People used A&E rather than their practice for a range of reasons, but the service that seemed likely to meet most people's needs was one that was available for long hours, at short notice, could assess their needs, and organize appropriate care/treatment/advice.

Quantitative research

Measurement of the outcomes of introducing a practice nurse triaging system showed less inappropriate A&E attendances; statistically significant findings, thus possibly generalizable.

Conclusions: A practice nurse triaging system can reduce inappropriate A&E attendance.

Mixed methods research

Studied the implementation of practice nurses offering a walk-in service to patients who did not have appointments. Quantified the number of attenders, length of appointments, outcomes of consultations, and number of inappropriate A&E attendances. Descriptive statistics were used and thus generalizability could not be commented on. Qualitative approaches were used to explore practice nurses' views of this service: nurses felt that the service was valuable, they needed some preparation and support in this role but gained confidence and soon felt able to assess and treat appropriately, found GPs and A&E useful resources in developing their skills knowledge and confidence. Some nurses had to reorganize their other commitments to cover the new hours, which was initially a problem.

Conclusions: Patients used the practice nurses' walk-in service and inappropriate A&E attendances were reduced. The qualitative findings suggested that the service was useful, but nurses needed preparation for and support in developing their role. Working with A&E on this was valuable. Changing their established working patterns was an important consideration for practice nurses.

Audit

An audit of a service where practice nurses offered patients the opportunity to phone between 9 and 11 each day and be advised of the best way to proceed. Identified how many calls were taken, the outcome of those calls, and the destination of the patients concerned, for example A&E, GP appointment, further advice from the practice nurse. Showed that a large number of calls were initially taken, but that these diminished over time. Initially, inappropriate A&E attendance was reduced, but began to rise again after three months.

Conclusions: This approach appeared to work well initially, but then declined. It seemed to work less well than the face-to-face contact seen in other studies.

Action research

Practice nurses developed an evening drop-in service between 7 and 9 pm, which was evaluated by measuring numbers of attendees, exploring the views of a group of patients who attended, and seeking staff feedback. The drop-in sessions were always fully used. Patients appreciated the out-of-hours timing of the service and lack of need for appointments. Nurses felt that although they had required some support at first with decision making, their confidence had developed over time with support from GPs and A&E staff (by telephone). The timing of the service required some negotiation and flexibility as the nurses and receptionists had not previously worked in the evenings. The service was initially offered two evenings a week, and expanded as staff became able to commit to shifts.

Conclusions: A practice nurse-led, out-of-hours drop-in service was useful, nurses needed support and preparation for this role, changes to existing hours of work needed to be planned for and negotiated.

Clinical guidelines
A guideline provided some useful information on how the service could be operationalized day to day.

Case reports and expert opinion
These provided some valuable insights into how the service could be set up and managed day to day.

Conclusion
From this evidence, Hannah proposed the development of a nurse-led triage service, which extended into the evening. She thought this would mean that practitioners and patients would have their preference for people being seen at the practice met, patients would feel able to disclose their actual needs, and would not encounter difficulties if they were unsure if these was urgent or not. Waiting times would be dependent on the numbers attending. Practitioners would be able to offer a service they felt was lacking, and would be less annoyed at patients using urgent appointment slots inappropriately. The practice nurses might also develop useful additional skills and knowledge.

The literature provided supporting evidence that this approach could work and could reduce inappropriate A&E attendance. It also indicated that there would be a value in face-to-face rather than telephone triaging. However, it would need planning, consideration of working hours and practices, and training, development and support for practitioners. These and the practicalities of setting the service up were things that Hannah would need to work on with her colleagues. She believed that the work would fit an action research approach.

Practice pointer 6.11

A key part of evaluating the evidence that will inform practice development is fitting together all the information gathered from different sources.

> **Activity 6.7**
>
> How could the sources of evidence available to you be used together to inform you in developing person-centred practice?

Summary

Hannah found a range of forms of evidence that would be useful to inform the developments in practice that she was considering. However, in order to keep the developments in practice person centred, this evidence had to be focused around the people for whom she intended to provide services, and their views, values and priorities. This meant that information on the views, priorities, opinions and perceptions of those receiving care were critical aspects of the evidence that would inform developments in practice. The views, experiences and perceptions of practitioners were also vital, as any developments in practice would need to be acceptable to them and practically viable.

Research, audit, evaluation, existing guidelines, expert opinion and case reports were among the other forms of evidence that Hannah thought would be useful. However, their quality and applicability to her particular practice area had to be evaluated before she decided whether or not they would be a useful part of her body of evidence. The various forms of evidence she had gathered then had to be integrated into a meaningful whole to determine the direction of developments in practice.

Having determined the way in which she thought practice could be developed, Hannah needed to decide how to go about introducing her ideas to her colleagues.

Case scenario

Nathan is the unit manager of a coronary care unit (CCU). He is looking to develop practice so that the unit works in a more person-centred way, and is exploring the different types of information he could use to assist him in this. In line with the principles of practice development methodology, he first wants to gain the perspectives of patients, their relatives and staff.

How could Nathan access information about what patients and their relatives think is good about the unit, and what could be improved?

Although Nathan could ask patients who are currently on the unit and their relatives what they think about provision, he does not think this would be the best approach. Because all the patients are acutely ill, often bordering on critically ill, they may not be best placed to consider the services they are receiving. They might also be concerned about the effect that any negative feedback could have on their care, which Nathan thinks would create a positively biased response. However, he wants to offer current patients and relatives the opportunity to provide feedback, and thinks that having comment, compliment and suggestion cards available for them to complete anonymously if they wish to may be useful in this respect.

To gain additional and potentially more in-depth information, Nathan is considering having discussions with ex-patients and their relatives, to hear their views and experiences of being on a CCU. He thinks this could be set up via invitations at follow-up clinics.

How could Nathan seek his colleagues' views on what is good, what works well, and what could be improved on the unit?

Nathan has considered holding discussions with the unit staff to ascertain their views. However, while he feels that he generally gets on well with everyone and is not seen as authoritarian, he is aware that he is the unit manager, with the perceived power issues that this naturally creates. People may be reluctant to criticize how things are, and fear repercussions if they suggest alterations in how the unit is run. He has considered distributing questionnaires that would provide staff with anonymity, but thinks these would end up focusing on specific technical elements of care, workload, rotas and suchlike. What he is really interested in is the culture of the unit and what this enables and inhibits in terms of person-centred care.

Having decided that neither of these options is ideal, Nathan is looking into setting up a series of reflective discussions for the unit staff, with a facilitator leading the process. The intention of these discussions will be to explore particular incidents or instances where a variety of factors, both positive and negative, have impacted on care provision. He believes that this may create an opportunity, arising from practice, for people to openly share their views. He has considered whether or not he should attend these discussions. On the one hand, he wonders if his presence will inhibit discussion. Conversely, he thinks that if he contributes to the discussion with what he feels is good as well as what could be improved in his own practice and that of the unit as a whole, others may feel more able to constructively discuss the way things are. He also believes that using this approach may be a good preparation for the later use of critical reflection, the focus of practice development methodology.

Nathan plans to augment these sources of information with naturally occurring informal conversations and observations in practice.

What are Nathan's views on the care provided in his workplace?

Nathan considers that the care provided on his unit is generally sound and technically efficient. The unit is always busy and patients often have to be sent to wards quickly to make room for another admission. This is not ideal, but pressure on beds is high. In theory, Nathan wants to be able to offer more person-centred care, but he struggles with how to achieve this in a busy, fast-moving service. He genuinely wants his team to help him explore this, because he does not have the answers. He thinks his team are, by and large, compassionate and often go the extra mile for patients and in particular relatives. However, this depends on the individuals concerned and the shift in question. Sometimes, if he is honest, it is hard to remain compassionate towards patients, relatives and his colleagues in a busy service with a fast patient turnover and many conflicting demands.

What could qualitative and quantitative research add to Nathan's knowledge about how his unit might develop practice?

Qualitative research could be useful for Nathan in providing evidence about how patients and relatives perceive and experience their time in a CCU and what matters to them. This might not be generalizable to his unit, but if in-depth descriptions are given of the context in which studies occur, he will be able to determine how transferable they are to his setting. Qualitative research may also provide him with valuable insights into the experiences of CCU staff, and what matters to them in their work. This could include what has helped other units to develop a more person-centred approach to care.

Quantitative research may be valuable in terms of providing statistical evidence about what generally adds to or detracts from patient, relative or staff satisfaction and the ability to deliver person-centred care. This might include measurements of changes in patient and staff satisfaction as a result of developing more person-centred care.

Nathan looked for systematic reviews about person-centred care in coronary care units at the Joanna Briggs Institute and the Cochrane Collaboration

Neither database had any systematic reviews directly related to what Nathan was interested in. They both had reviews in their databases that might be useful to revisit if the unit decided to implement any specific interventions within the general concept of person-centred care.

Nathan thought that the lack of systematic reviews was probably because there was relatively little research in this area, which would render a systematic review unlikely. In addition, Cochrane reviews generally investigate the effects of interventions for prevention, treatment and rehabilitation, and assess the accuracy of diagnostic tests for a given condition in a specific patient group and setting (www.cochrane.org/cochrane-reviews). This meant that the type of information Nathan was seeking was unlikely to be found there.

What might case reports and expert opinions add to Nathan's knowledge about developing practice in his workplace?

Case reports could give Nathan an important insight into what individual patients and relatives had felt or experienced during their CCU stays, what mattered to them, and what contributed to their perspectives. A case report of any unit that had tried to develop more person-centred care would be useful for him to get ideas from. Similarly, expert opinion or experiences might be useful, especially if they dealt with how to develop person-centred care on a CCU.

Although the findings from these sources of evidence would not be generalizable, they could provide Nathan with some valuable insights, ideas and contact details of people who had been involved in the type of development he was planning.

How could the sources of evidence available to Nathan be used together to inform the development of person-centred practice?

Nathan thought that the experiences and perceptions of practitioners, patients and relatives of patients from his unit would need to be the focus of the evidence used to develop practice, because these related directly to the context and situation in question. His own reflections and views would also be important, particularly as he was the unit manager, with some influence in the unit and on how others might perceive things. Although he intended the emphasis to be on evidence from the unit itself, any research, case studies and expert opinions Nathan could find would add to what he discovered from within his own unit, and would give useful insights into what might work for them, what might not, and why this might be. They might confirm and add weight to the evidence from his own unit, or might challenge this evidence, and give him and his team ideas about alternatives.

Additional resources

www.casp-uk.net/#!casp-tools-checklists/c18f8
Provides guidance and checklists for evaluating a variety of studies.

http://joannabriggs.org
www.thecochranelibrary.com/view/0/index.html
Provide access to details of systematic reviews that have been carried out, and resources about how systematic reviews are conducted.

www.medicine.ox.ac.uk/bandolier
Bandolier houses a range of materials about evidence-based health.

Practice Development and Change 7

Chapter overview

- Understanding the principles of managing change can be useful in facilitating the processes required to develop person-centred practice.
- Practice development methodology focuses on people, and understanding the people aspects of change can be especially relevant to developing person-centred practice. This includes exploring the things that contribute to people resisting change, such as feelings of loss, lack of confidence in working in a new way, competing priorities and time factors.
- Determining how to reduce the forces that may restrain the development of person-centred practice, while also increasing the forces that will drive it, can be useful. This incorporates identifying how ready people are for change, and how key stakeholders and opinion leaders will influence other people's adoption of a new way of working.

Clare is the manager of a house for adults with moderate to severe learning disabilities. The house is located within a complex that includes a daycare area and a respite care facility. Clare is planning to use the principles of practice development methodology to work with her team on developing a more person-centred approach to care. She is now thinking about the practical steps she will need to take to encourage her team to want to work in a more person-centred way, and believes that some of the principles of change management may be useful to guide her in this.

Change and practice development

Developing practice requires people to alter something about the way they work. Depending on the approach adopted, this may be practical aspects of their work or their attitudes, values and priorities (McCormack 2006). As Chapters 2 and 3 identified, practice development methodology focuses on facilitating a more person-centred approach to care, rather than altering particular practical aspects of care provision (McCormack et al. 2007, King and Kelly 2011). Clare has identified some areas where she thinks her team could work in a more person-centred way, such as the timing of daily activities and how residents' interests are provided for in their living spaces and recreational activities. However, rather than focusing on particular elements of care, she wants to help her team move to a more person-centred ethos in everything they do. Clare aims to use the tools described in Chapter 4, such as individual and group reflection and critical companionship, to enable staff to think about what they do, how they work and how person centred this is. However, to begin this process, she will need to persuade people to make the initial effort to engage in considering and discussing how they work and whether they want to change this. This is where she feels that the principles of managing change can help her.

Practice pointer 7.1

- Developing practice involves changing something about how things are done at present.
- Developing person-centred practice means changing things so that a more person-centred approach to care is developed.
- The principles of managing change can be useful for effecting some elements of developing person-centred practice.

Practice development methodology focuses on the personhood of those cared for and those doing the caring. It also recognizes the effects that the culture, social circumstances and history of those involved, as individuals and groups, have on situations, and how the level of power people feel they have impacts on what they do. Similarly, managing change successfully requires a great deal of attention to be paid to what a particular change will mean to the individuals concerned, and how the groups they belong to will influence this. Austin and Currie (2003) and McLean (2011) describe two aspects of suggestions to alter the way people work, which may influence their acceptance of it. They term these 'change' and 'transition'. In this context, change refers to the observable things that happen or need to be done differently. If Clare asks her team to meet to reflect on their practice every Tuesday afternoon, the change will be that on Tuesday afternoons they all assemble to do this, instead of engaging in another activity. Transition concerns the emotional or psychological elements of change: what people feel, experience and see as important about it. It concerns how people would feel about meeting to review their practice, and might include:

- their experiences of what happened the last time they were asked to revisit their way of working

- whether they see this as potentially valuable or a threat
- how the individuals concerned and the group as a whole manage their feelings.

The change in what has to be done may be relatively straightforward, but if the transition for the individuals involved is significant, considerable effort is likely to be required to achieve the alteration in practice.

Unless people are willing to engage in the process of developing more person-centred practice, it will not work, however well planned and organized the processes intended to facilitate it are. So, Clare can see that she will need to introduce the idea of developing practice in a way that makes the transitional elements of it as positive as possible.

Practice pointer 7.2

- Change involves the practical, visible aspects of working in a new way, but also how people perceive and feel about the proposed changes.
- How people feel about changing the ethos of their work is critical to the development of person-centred practice.

Practice pointer 7.3

Practice development methodology focuses on people. Managing change effectively also needs to be focused on the people involved, and how change affects them as individuals and teams.

Engaging people in developing practice

Chin and Benne (1985) identify three approaches to motivating people to change their practice: the empirical rational, normative re-educative and power coercive approaches.

The empirical rational approach

The empirical rational approach (Chin and Benne 1985) assumes that people will alter the way they work if they understand the reason for doing so and consider it to be in their own or the general best interests. It therefore focuses on enabling people to understand why a new way of doing things is being suggested and presenting convincing evidence to support this (McLean 2011). Clare thinks that this will be important, as people will need to understand why she is suggesting that they revisit the way they work (Paton and McCalman

2008, Ludwick and Doucette 2009, Hall and Hord 2011). This will include outlining the possible benefits that using a more person-centred approach may bring for residents and staff. How this information is delivered, as well as the message itself, will, however, be influential in whether or not people are enthused to alter their approach to care (Parkin 2009: 159–60).

Oakland and Tanner (2007) and Cameron and Green (2009) suggest that people are more likely to embrace change if it builds on the positive aspects of their existing situation. Clare has come across the principles of appreciative inquiry, as described in Chapter 4, and thinks they will be useful in this respect. Appreciative inquiry is based on building on the strengths of individuals, teams and organizations and what they do well, rather than focusing on what is seen as problematic (Moore 2008, Parish 2012). Clare believes that using this approach will enable her to focus on instances where she has seen her colleagues working in a person-centred way, and to present her idea as exploring how they can build on and develop this existing good practice. She hopes this will encourage individuals, and the team as a whole, to become collaborators with her in developing the positive elements of their practice, rather than seeing person-centred practice as her idea, which she is imposing on them.

In addition to understanding why developing a more person-centred approach to care is being suggested, Clare believes that her team will want to know about the practicalities of what they are being asked to do (Giangreco and Peccei 2005, Golden 2006, McLean 2011, Paré et al. 2011). This will include what engaging in the process of reflection (as described in Chapter 4) will require of them, but also the practical details of what will happen: when meetings will take place, how long they will last, and how those who cannot attend will be catered for.

While how the initial idea about developing person-centred practice is delivered will be important, Clare will also need to restate this information from time to time as messages can easily be misinterpreted, distorted or forgotten (Schifalacqua et al. 2009, Hall and Hord 2011). Although she intends to focus on building on and valuing what her team does well, Clare knows that it will be easy for the message to be translated into it being a fault-finding exercise. Thus, her ongoing communication and actions need to confirm that the intention is to concentrate on how the team can develop elements of existing good practice, rather than emphasizing deficiencies in care that need to be corrected.

While Clare thinks the empirical rational approach will be important, she does not believe it will be enough to convince her team to engage in the process of developing person-centred care. Although it will enable her to outline the perceived benefits of this way of working, these will have to outweigh any disadvantages or threats that staff may feel a person-centred approach will bring (Erwin and Garman 2010). She thinks her main focus will therefore need to be on the normative re-educative approach.

The normative re-educative approach

The normative re-educative approach (Chin and Benne 1985) focuses on the social and cultural implications of change and explores why people may or may not favour a new way of working, regardless of its apparent worth. It links with the need to consider the transitional elements of change and is consistent with practice development methodology's acknowledgment of the complexity of people, and the interactions between individuals and their social context.

The normative re-educative approach also considers it necessary for people to own, take an active part in and control the development of a new way of working in order for it to be successfully introduced (Ludwick and Doucette 2009). This fits with the ethos of practice development methodology, whose underpinning links with critical social theory and critical realism include the empowerment of individuals and groups (Bevan et al. 2012, Oliver 2012). Change is often described as coming from the bottom up (initiated by front-line staff) or top down (initiated and directed by management, and required of frontline staff) (Hall and Hord 2011). The ethos of practice development methodology is most consistent with bottom-up approaches, where change is owned, developed and controlled by those most closely concerned with its practical implementation (Chin and Hamer 2006). This fits with the normative re-educative approach to change, which requires practitioners to feel personally inspired to work in a different way, rather than this being imposed on them (McCormack et al. 2013). It is also an important part of enabling people to become collaborators in the process of changing practice, rather than change being owned and driven by the person leading it. Clare's intention is to work with staff in a way that enables them to determine, and have control of, the aspects of their work they change. To achieve this, she plans to use a reflective approach, which enables people to identify what they already do well and want to build on. So, she thinks that using the normative re-educative approach to change will fit the ethos of what she is trying to introduce and be a vital part of getting people to buy in to working in a more person-centred way.

The power coercive approach

The power coercive approach to change is not something Clare wants to use. In this approach, power of one kind or another is used to achieve change, and fear of the consequences of doing or not doing something, rather than the intrinsic value of the new way of working, drives people to comply. People are motivated to change by behavioural means (such as positive or negative reinforcement), not because of the intrinsic benefits or rewards of developing practice (Cameron and Green 2009). The power coercive approach also focuses on particular behaviours, processes or events, which contrasts with the focus of practice development methodology on exploring the beliefs, values and priorities that underpin practice. In addition, Clare thinks that a coercive approach is incompatible with emancipation and transformation – the ethos of practice development methodology – and will not encourage people to see themselves as collaborators in a joint process of developing practice. Pragmatically, she considers the power coercive approach inappropriate, as it will be impossible for her to tell her colleagues to be more person centred. The only way to achieve this will be to work with them so that, as individuals and a group, they understand what person-centredness is and want to achieve this.

Practice pointer 7.4

Chin and Benne's (1985) three approaches to change are empirical rational, normative re-educative and power coercive.

Activity 7.1

How would you use the empirical rational, normative re-educative and power coercive approaches to change to introduce the idea of working in a more person-centred way in your workplace?

Having considered the general approaches to introducing new practice that she wants to adopt, Clare is looking at the normative re-educative approach in more detail, so as to identify what might encourage, or detract from, people embracing the idea of working in a more person-centred way. First, she is considering how she will know whether or not people are supportive of her suggestion to work in a more person-centred way.

How person-centred care might be opposed

People being disinclined to work in a new way is often described as 'resistance to change', and linked with the idea of open opposition to innovations. However, resistance to change may also be passive, where people do not openly oppose a new way of working, but have no intention of altering what they do, and may sabotage other people's attempts to do so. This can be equally, if not more, difficult to overcome than overt resistance (Parkin 2009). Clare thinks this may be a significant form of resistance to developing person-centred care, as her colleagues are less likely to openly oppose the idea as to find ways to avoid engaging in the process.

Another important form of resistance is apathy, where an idea is not really opposed but is not considered important enough for people to make an effort to engage with it (Giangreco and Peccei 2005). Clare thinks this may be a major factor for her: she believes that many of her team will, in principle, agree that working in a more person-centred way is a good idea, but she is less certain that it will be seen as a day-to-day priority that is important enough to really make an effort for. She will, therefore, need to move beyond giving information, as seen in the empirical rational approach, to motivating people to think that this is sufficiently important to take the time and effort to achieve (Ludwick and Doucette 2009, Paré et al. 2011). There are also a couple of staff who Clare thinks will probably see this idea as the latest fad and will believe that if they do nothing, it will soon be forgotten (Parkin 2009). They will probably not think it is worth arguing about, but simply ignore it, assuming that if they do so it will go away.

Whether resistance is passive or active, thinking carefully about what may be causing it is important, because what people say may not reflect what they really mean, are concerned about, or do.

Practice pointer 7.5

Passive resistance and apathy can be the most difficult forms of resistance to change to manage.

Change and loss

One reason why people may not engage in a new way of working is the losses that they feel, or fear, it will bring (Price 2008, Hall and Hord 2011). Moving to a more person-centred approach to care is likely to change the way people in Clare's team work, feel relatively confident with, and can easily achieve on a day-to-day basis. The house currently runs quite smoothly and is well ordered, with routines and processes that everyone knows and accepts. Exactly what will happen if they move to a more person-centred approach is unknown, which is likely to engender feelings of insecurity, loss of familiarity and loss of control (Giangreco and Peccei 2005, Hall and Hord 2011). Established routines and how things are done are likely to alter, which may create feelings of loss for familiar structures, processes and control of situations (Grol and Grimshaw 2003, Hall and Hord 2011). It may also mean that the house does not run as predictably and smoothly as it currently does, with a risk that things that are now part of established routines will be forgotten. Clare thinks that an important part of minimizing the losses people feel or fear will be to emphasize that the plan is for the team to move reflectively, one step at a time, in their quest to develop person-centred care. For instance, a starting point may be to begin to engage in conversations to elicit what residents are interested in, rather than changing particular routines or events that could threaten people's sense of security.

Practice pointer 7.6

Change can create feelings of loss, and understanding these can help to identify why change may be resisted.

Activity 7.2

What losses might working in a more person-centred way bring for people in your team?

Change can alter the status of individuals or groups (Parkin 2009). This may relate to formal roles and status or informal but nonetheless important roles, such as how people are viewed, and the perceptions they and others have of their knowledge, expertise, skills or connections (Carroll and Quijada 2004). Clare knows, for instance, that some staff are seen as the best at organizing recreational activities for residents. If a more person-centred approach is adopted, with more individualized activities, these people may feel a threat to their informal expert roles. Clare thinks that focusing the process of developing practice on what people already do well may be useful in addressing such feelings. This will enable reflective discussions to include how people's existing strengths and skills can be used in any developments. For instance, by using the critical creativity that is a part of practice development methodology (Manley et al. 2013a), the acknowledged experts in organizing activities could be encouraged to help others to creatively imagine what might be set up for individual residents.

Loss has been associated with people having to rewrite their personal and corporate narratives and find a place for their history and memories in the new order of things (Krueger 2006). Similarly, change may mean that individuals and groups have to review their personal and corporate narratives and find meaning and a place for what they have done, valued and been valued for in the past. Clare thinks that an important part of enabling people to move to a more person-centred way of working will be to help them to find benefits, a place for themselves and links with what they value, in the new way of working (Price 2008, McLean 2011). By using the principles of appreciative inquiry, what is currently good about the team and their work will be the initial focus, with the intention being to develop this and take it with them as they develop more person-centred care.

Nonetheless, Clare will need to be alert to individuals and the team as a whole feeling a sense of loss for what they have been and have valued. This may include not only skills and status, but more general issues such as the day being organized so that staff can spend informal time together when the residents are all watching TV. This is currently an important part of their camaraderie and enables them to work well as a team. Clare thinks that she will need to stress that practice development methodology includes a recognition of the personhood of staff, and to encourage people to think about and discuss how altering the way they work will affect them. This will require reflective discussions to be open, respectful and nonjudgmental, so that staff can talk about themselves as people with needs, priorities, values and beliefs.

Practice pointer 7.7

Change can create feelings of loss of:

* security, familiarity and control
* roles and responsibilities
* perceived expertise and confidence
* personal and team history
* what has been achieved and valued.

Activity 7.3

What good things about your workplace's current practice would you be able to incorporate into an ongoing narrative of person-centred care?

Confidence in person-centred caring

Clare is enthusiastic about adopting a more person-centred approach to care and thinks it is in line with good practice. However, she knows that others may have different perspectives. It will be important, therefore, that discussions include the expectation that people should raise any concerns they have about this innovation. As well as this being a part of the ethos of person-centred practice development, in which everyone's views are valued, encouraging people to raise concerns is an important part of developing effective practice. If no one questions, or feels able to question, a new idea, its possible pitfalls or problems may be missed (McDonnell et al. 2006). So, although Clare may find challenges to her ideas about developing more person-centred care off-putting, they may also make any new way of working more robust in the long term (Fronda and Moriceau 2008, Wright 2010).

Practice pointer 7.8

Resistance to change can be useful: it enables questions to be asked, assumptions to be challenged and pitfalls to be considered. This often makes developments in practice more robust in the long term.

People's acceptance of changes in practice are often influenced by their confidence in their ability to work in the new way. If individuals feel uncertain of their ability to perform activities in which they are currently confident and competent, it is likely to detract from their enthusiasm to work in a new way, even if they can see why it would, in principle, be beneficial (Cameron and Green 2009). Clare's colleagues may truly think that enabling residents to engage in more individualized activities is a good idea. However, if they are not sure that they can provide these, they may oppose the idea, or decide each day that they will do it tomorrow, until eventually it is forgotten. Clare thinks that people being supported by a critical companion (as discussed in Chapter 4), who can challenge but also encourage and support them daily as they attempt to change the way they work, will be useful in this respect.

Some members of Clare's team may also feel uncomfortable about the reflective activities that are a key part of practice development methodology, especially if they are unfamiliar with this approach. Assurances that they will be supported in the process, and that blame or criticism are not the aim, alongside evidence that this is the reality of how discussions unfold, will probably be necessary to convince some people to participate.

Clare thinks that an important part of allaying any concerns her team have about developing person-centred care may be to clarify that the idea is supported by higher level managers (Allan 2007). Her intention is to use a bottom-up approach to change, in which frontline practitioners determine and own their direction of travel. Nonetheless, it will be useful for them to know that managerial staff support them in this and will not be critical of the outcomes of their attempts to develop person-centred practice. It will, however, be necessary for Clare to achieve the balance between providing assurances of managerial support and implying that this is something that is required, and being monitored, by those in authority.

Practice pointer 7.9

Although practice development methodology focuses on bottom-up approaches to change, it is also important to have, and be known to have, managerial support for and engagement with it.

> ## Activity 7.4
>
> What aspects of working in a more person-centred way might cause your colleagues concern?

Time

People not having, or not perceiving themselves to have, the time to do things differently is often cited as a reason why change does not happen (Oxman and Flottorp 2001, Grol and Grimshaw 2003). Clare's colleagues may feel that they do not have the time to engage in reflective activities or discussions about their work. Equally, when particular changes in how people work are suggested, these may be considered too time-consuming to do, even if they seem a good idea. For example, facilitating individual activities for residents may be seen as more time-consuming than holding a group activity, despite being a good idea in principle. Clare realizes that she will need to constantly check whether people perceive time to be a barrier to them achieving person-centred care. By being alert to this possibility, she will be able to creatively and supportively explore with individuals or groups how time-related barriers to working in a more person-centred way might be overcome.

Clare also believes that she will need to be alert to a lack of time being used as an argument for person-centred care not being achievable, when the real reason is other factors, such as the losses people are feeling, or it not being seen as a priority. She thinks that critical companionship and reflective discussions will be useful in this respect, as they will enable people to be supportively challenged to explore the actual reasons why they do not seem to have enough time to provide person-centred care.

> ### Practice pointer 7.10
>
> * Lack of time can be a barrier to people adopting change.
> * It may be necessary to explore whether time being perceived as a barrier masks other reasons for people not participating in a new way of working.

Workplace culture and history

As well as individual concerns, the culture and history of a workplace are likely to influence how the people in it respond to suggestions for change (Parkin 2009, McCabe 2010, Hall and Hord 2011). This includes the way in which the group as a whole have experienced change in the past, but also individuals' experiences of change. Clare is aware that her team seldom change or challenge how they work, and that people are unlikely to be confident in questioning their practice and using reflective activities. At the same time, because the team has not tried this approach before, there is no negative history to influence their perceptions of it. Equally, while there is no corporate history of this approach being used, individuals may have previous personal experiences, unrelated to their present employment, which will influence their views.

The culture of Clare's workplace is very much that it is a happy place, where the staff get on well. There is a lot of good-humoured banter at work and people do not take life too seriously. These are aspects of their culture that people will be unlikely to want to lose. The residents are usually treated well, although care is somewhat ritualized and events generally happen en masse. However, the general feeling is that this is a necessary compromise in order to get everything done. The team ethos is based on this premise and, as far as Clare knows, has been accepted as such for many years. Challenging this may be problematic, and is one reason why Clare aims to introduce the idea of developing what people are good at and value as a step to developing more person-centred care. For instance, she thinks that recognizing the strength of practitioners seeing each other as individuals who matter will enable her to introduce the idea of this valuing of people being extended to how residents are viewed.

Practice pointer 7.11

- Practice development methodology views a workplace's culture and history as important.
- A workplace's culture and history are likely to influence how individuals and groups respond to change.

Clare has identified several ways in which using the normative re-educative approach to change will be beneficial in addressing things that might detract from her team achieving more person-centred care. However, whether the things that will drive the process will be outweighed by those that may detract from it is something she now needs to consider. These are the forces that drive or restrain change.

Driving and restraining forces in change

The things that are likely to positively affect change are sometimes described as 'driving forces', or facilitators of change, and those that will inhibit change as 'restraining forces' (Lewin 1951, Parkin 2009). Weighing these up and determining how strong each side of the equation is has been described as 'force field analysis' (Lewin 1951). For change to succeed, the overall driving force needs to outweigh the restraining force. The driving and restraining forces may be related to each other, or unrelated, but the overall strength needs to be positive for change to happen. The stronger the positive force, theoretically at least, the less problematic introducing new practice will be.

If the forces driving a change do not sufficiently outweigh the restraining forces, something needs to alter before an innovation can succeed. The ideal is to reduce the restraining forces and increase the driving forces. However, of the two actions, finding ways to reduce the restraining forces is usually the more vital. If the driving forces are increased without addressing the restraining forces, the tension between the two increases (Iles and Cranfield 2004). If the negative forces are reduced, there is likely to be less resistance to the force of change, which creates a smoother pathway.

The factors that make up driving and restraining forces may be the people factors described in the normative re-educative approach to change, or practical issues. Clare's aim is to change her workplace culture to being more person centred, so the people factors are likely to be the most crucial (Grol and Grimshaw 2003, Paton and McCalman 2008). However, the practicalities required to achieve this are also vital because without these, however strongly motivated people are to participate in a new way of working, it will be impossible.

In most situations, a percentage of people will be fairly indifferent about any new way of working (Giangreco and Peccei 2005). This group will probably follow the path of least resistance in terms of whether or not to participate, so making the new way of working as easy as possible to achieve increases the chance of them taking part. In Clare's case, making reflective sessions easy to attend will encourage those who are indifferent to do so. If it is difficult to attend, those who are relatively apathetic will opt out and those who are disinclined will have an excuse not to participate. Thus, having a room available to meet in and everyone being free to attend will probably be as important as presenting the information about developing person-centredness in an appealing way.

Considering the forces that are likely to drive and restrain the introduction of more person-centred working, particularly the human factors, has led Clare to think about how ready individuals and groups within her team are likely to be to engage in this process.

Activity 7.5

What would be likely to drive or restrain developing a more person-centred way of working in your team?

Practice pointer 7.12

For change to succeed, the overall force driving change needs to be stronger than the restraining force.

Readiness for change

Readiness for change has been described as the extent to which individuals and groups are inclined to accept, in principle, and then adopt a new way of working (Paré et al. 2011). This is usually seen as existing on a continuum, from being ready to change (high readiness for change) to not being ready to participate in change (low readiness for change) (Holt et al. 2007, Paré et al. 2011). Weiner et al. (2008) suggest that readiness for change includes structural elements, such as the resources that are needed, and psychological elements – people's attitudes, beliefs and intentions. Other writers describe how readiness for change includes people's cognitive acceptance of change – whether they think it is, in theory, a good idea – and their emotional acceptance of change – whether it is something they feel willing and able to engage in (Paré et al. 2011). These aspects of readiness for change are not always easy to separate and can become attributed to one another. For instance, someone may claim that a structural element, such as being too busy, makes it impossible for them to engage in reflective discussions, even if the real reason is a psychological element such as them feeling threatened by the idea.

Clare thinks it will be useful for her to reflect on how ready individuals in her team are likely to be to consider working in a more person-centred way, so that she can assess how this might influence the forces that drive or restrain change. Prochaska and DiClemente's (1992) model of readiness for change describes the stages of readiness as pre-contemplation, contemplation, determination to change, action, and maintenance of new practice. Although this work is based on changing personal behaviour, not professional practice, it can still be a useful framework within which to consider readiness for new practice.

Practice pointer 7.13

Prochaska and DiClemente's (1992) stages of readiness for change are:

* pre-contemplation
* contemplation
* determination to change
* action
* maintenance of new practice.

---

1 *Pre-contemplation:* People are not contemplating, or willing to contemplate, change. They are either unaware that change might be suggested, or are aware of proposals for change but are not prepared to consider these. If the majority of the people concerned are at this stage, something has to

happen before things can move forward. Clare suspects that almost all her team are at this stage at present, as they seem happy with how they work and are probably not thinking about changing it. However, she also thinks it unlikely that they will be opposed to the idea of more person-centred working: they are simply not aware that it is a possibility. She believes that when she introduces the idea, most people will at least move to the contemplation stage.

2 *Contemplation stage*: Here, people have moved beyond dismissing the idea of change and are thinking about it and weighing up its pros and cons. They have not decided they will participate, but it is a possibility. Clare hopes that the majority of her team will move to this stage. However, for some, the contemplation stage may be followed by a return to the pre-contemplation stage, if they decide that this way of working is not something they want to participate in.

3 *Determination to change*: Preparation for change is a stage Clare hopes the majority of her team will move to. At this point, individuals have decided they are ready and willing to participate in a new way of working. For Clare, this will be reached when people decide that person-centred care is a good idea, worth pursuing, and show a genuine commitment to engaging in reflective activities related to their own practice.

4 *Action:* Changing is the stage at which people who are prepared to change engage in the actual process of changing the way things are. In Clare's team, this will be where people attend and engage in individual and group reflection, work effectively with a critical companion, and actively seek to be more person centred in their day-to-day work.

5 *Maintaining change:* Prochaska and DiClemente's (1992) fifth or final stage of change. Chapter 10 discusses in more detail the processes and challenges of sustaining person-centred practice, but if attention is not given to this stage, all the work put into the preceding stages will often be wasted.

Readiness for change can be seen in individual and team or organizational terms: how ready individuals, teams or organizations are to adopt a new way of working. Critical social theory and critical realism, which underpin practice development methodology, see individuals as a part of their social and cultural contexts, and consider the effects that groups and society as a whole have on individual actions and perceptions (Freeman and Vasconcelos 2010, Bevan et al. 2012, Lapum et al. 2012, Oliver 2012). How ready individuals within the team, but also the team as a whole, are for change and the way each person or group is likely to influence others are all important considerations for Clare. This means she needs to consider not only who within the team might be at each stage of readiness for change, but also how, and to what degree, each person or group of people might influence others.

Key stakeholders and opinion leaders

When a new way of working is suggested, the influence that individual people have on a group as a whole can be critical to the success of the proposed innovation. This may be because key individuals support the idea, and inspire others to do so, or because they are opposed to it and hold others back. How individual readiness for change will affect the readiness of others is, therefore, an important consideration for Clare (Qian and Daniels 2008, Cameron and Green 2009, Erwin and Garman 2010).

Opinion leaders are the people in a group who are listened to and whose opinions carry more weight than anyone else's (Iles and Cranfield 2004). They may not be high-profile people but, for one reason or another, they have extra influence (Hall and Hord 2011). People may be opinion leaders because they are well respected and turned to when expert advice is needed (Hall and Horde 2011). Equally, they may be people whose opinion counts because of their personality or history in the organization. Because their views influence others, they can significantly help or hinder the develop-ment of person-centred care (Iles and Cranfield 2004, Richens et al. 2004). Clare thinks she knows who the main opinion leaders in her team are. There are two people who have worked in the house for longer than anyone else, have seen many changes come and go, and can be relied on to advise others as to whether they should pay any attention to a new idea or concern. They are often invaluable, because they keep the numerous reports and rumours of change the workplace is exposed to in perspective. The downside is that if they see a new idea as simply the latest fad, they will easily discourage others from taking it seriously. There is also a member of staff who is enthusiastic about organizing group activities and events for the residents. She is well liked, charismatic and her views on a move to more person-centred care will almost certainly influence those of others.

As well as those whose opinion counts most, it is important to identify the major stakeholders in any change (Parkin 2009, Schifalacqua et al. 2009). Stakeholders are those who stand to gain or lose something because of a new way of working. As identified previously, gains and losses can include people's informal status, perception of self and security, and these considerations are likely to be important for Clare in considering what is at stake for each indi-vidual in her team. For example, the member of staff who is good at organ-izing group activities may well stand to lose her unofficial role as the best activities' organizer if care and activities become more personalized. She is a key stakeholder, as well as an opinion leader.

Having identified who the key stakeholders are, it is also useful to think about how much power each one has and how much their desire to see change enacted or failing will influence others and the process as a whole (Parkin

2009). This can be managerial power, although stakeholders may have no offi-cial power, but the equally strong power of influence. The key stakeholder Clare has identified has no official power, but is likely to have considerable power of influence.

Practice pointer 7.14

Opinion leaders and key stakeholders are important influences on whether or not change is successfully adopted

---

Activity 7.6

Who are the key opinion leaders and stakeholders in your team?

To successfully implement a new way of working, a critical mass who are ready to work in the new way are generally needed (Cameron and Green 2009, Hall and Hord 2011). One of the challenges involved in managing change is that while some people will be enthusiastic at the outset and will remain so, others will not be and will take some time to come on board (Hall and Hord 2011). Keeping the enthusiasts on board, being aware of those who may be wavering and knowing who is likely to influence them, while trying to increase the number and strength of those who support the initiative is part of the juggling process of managing change (Golden 2006, Reinhardt and Keller 2009).

The usual pattern of people adopting change can be represented by a bell curve, where support for innovation starts slowly, gradually picks up speed, then flattens off, with a final few people coming on board late in the process (Hall and Hord 2011). In any change, there are likely to be 'innovators', who initiate the change or are keen for it to take place (in this case, Clare), and 'early adopters', who agree with the idea for change and create the impetus required to carry it forward. These groups, who essentially lead the change, are followed by what are known as the 'early majority', who adopt change as they see others accepting it, and the 'late majority', who initially reject the change, but conform when everyone else seems to be participating. The final group are the 'laggards', who continue to reject change, either forever or until the new way of doing things becomes established practice (Rogers 1995, Hall and Hord 2011).

People who are at different stages in adopting change are likely to influ-ence each other. Clare's intention is to make this work to her advantage by harnessing the commitment of those who embrace the idea of person-centred practice to bring others on board, rather than allowing the laggards to derail to process (Hall and Hord 2011). To achieve this, she needs the most influential people on board at the outset or in the early stages of the process. Knowing who they are will assist her to introduce the idea of person-centred care in a way that particularly encourages them to be, or to become, enthusiastic about it.

Although those who oppose a new way of working can be disruptive to the process, if they do not represent a significant force, it is useful to avoid becoming preoccupied with them to the detriment of maintaining the enthusiasm of those who are on board (Hall and Hord 2011). Clare thinks that identifying who is likely to oppose the idea of person-centred working will enable her to consider who they may influence and the probable effect of their influence, so that she can devote appropriate, but not excessive time to managing any resistance they show.

Practice pointer 7.15

The usual pattern of people adopting change:

• Innovators initiate the change or are keen for it to take place.
• Early adopters agree with the idea for change and create the impetus required to carry it forward.
• Early majority adopt change as they see others accepting it.
• Late majority initially reject the change, but eventually conform when everyone else seems to be doing so.
• Laggards continue to reject change, forever or until the new way of doing things becomes established practice.

Planning

Practice development methodology is evolutionary, with activities predicated largely on how individuals decide they should take their practice forward. However, the process still requires some planning. As well as looking into the people factors associated with introducing more person-centred care, Clare is also checking the practicalities of what needs to be done. This includes the people, steps and resources that will be needed to begin the process of developing practice, and when key events will happen (Hall and Hord 2011). Thinking through this level of detail makes it less likely that she will miss anything and should mean that any practical barriers to people participating will be anticipated and overcome.

A vital part of planning any change is determining the resources that will be needed and how they will be secured (Macphee and Suryaprakash 2010,

Hall and Hord 2011). This includes making sure that everything that is needed for the new way of working is available and that there is enough of it (NICE 2007, Paton and McCalman 2008). In Clare's case, a time and place for the team to meet and discuss the idea of developing more person-centred practice and for ongoing reflective discussions will be needed. As Clare thinks it will be useful to use an external facilitator for reflective discussions and to work with individuals as a critical companion, she has had to decide who this will be and how funding for their services will work.

Deciding on the timescale for change is useful, so that those leading change and those being asked to participate know what is expected to happen, and when it is expected to happen (Schifalacqua et al. 2009). For Clare, this involves planning when she will hold the initial information-giving meetings, how long each meeting will take, when and how she will aim to engage people in reflective work, and how and when she will introduce and implement the idea of 'critical companionship'.

Planning any change includes determining whether people will need to gain any additional skills or knowledge (Golden 2006, NICE 2007, Hall and Hord 2011). If they will, how these skills will be acquired and whether they will need to be assessed should be considered (NICE 2007). It is also useful to think about whether any necessary education or training will be seen as a driving or restraining force, for example an opportunity to acquire new and useful skills, or a drain on people's valuable time. Clare thinks her colleagues will probably need to develop their skills and confidence in reflecting on their work. However, this will be a part of the practice development process, not a separate activity.

It can be useful to have a plan or timetable to document and monitor the practical events that are required in order to develop practice, so as to make sure that everything that needs to be done is done and to help keep things on track. Clare also thinks that being able to show people when concrete events will happen and why they are needed will reduce any uncertainty they feel, but also emphasize that this is not an abstract idea that will soon pass. Her plan for introducing a more person-centred approach to care is shown in Table 7.1.

Nonetheless, plans need to be flexible: if one goal gets delayed, then other dates may need to be altered in light of this. It is usually better to replan than to try and do an impossible catch-up task, become disheartened and give up. The key aim for Clare is to enable her team to move towards a more person-centred approach to care. She wants to keep this at the centre of all her considerations and be flexible about timing and progress, rather than trying to rush to meet goals at the cost of enabling people to engage in in-depth reflection and discussion. However, her plan gives her a good starting point from which to work.

Table 7.1 Plan for introducing a more person-centred approach to care

Action	Person/people leading	Resources needed	Date
Meet with whole team to discuss developing more person-centred approach to care: four episodes to capture as many staff as possible	Clare	Room, adequate staffing	1 May 2014, 14:00–15:00 2 May 2014, 14:00–15:00 6 May 2014, 14:00–15:00 7 May 2014, 14:00–15:00
Email information to whole team: to follow up information given at meetings, pick up on points raised, and for anyone not able to attend	Clare	Time, access to computer	9 May 2014
Facilitator to meet informally with staff to explain how reflective activities will be organized and run	Clare and Joanne (facilitator)	Room, adequate staffing, funding for Joanne's time	2 June 2014, 14:00–15:00 6 June 2014, 14:00–15:00
Begin one-on-one reflective sessions with facilitator	Joanne	Rotas to match Joanne's availability with individual staff availability, adequate staffing levels to release individuals, funding for Joanne's time	9 June onwards: aim for Joanne to meet all staff by the end of July
Begin reflective group activities	Joanne and Clare (Clare to organize practicalities)	Adequate staffing, room, funding for Joanne's time	1 August 2014
Discuss using critical companionship at reflective group meeting	Joanne and Clare (Clare to organize practicalities)	Adequate staffing, room, funding for Joanne's time	1 September 2014

While Clare hopes that the development of person-centred practice will become a collaborative team effort, she is aware that achieving this may take time. Her planning therefore includes identifying people who work in other parts of the complex that the house is located within from whom she may be able to gain peer support and collaborate with. She believes this will assist her in maintaining her enthusiasm, resolve and vision (Lothian 2005). Clare is also considering how she can communicate and collaborate with people who are interested or engaged in developing person-centred care nationally and internationally. To this end, she is looking at publications, blogs, discussion forums, conferences and special interest groups where she may be able to meet like-minded people. She hopes that these avenues will enable her to exchange ideas about the ideals of person-centred care, how to implement this in practice and gain peer support and encouragement (Lothian 2005).

Activity 7.7

What practical resources would you need to develop person-centred care in your workplace?

Summary

Change alters the status quo, creates uncertainty about what people are expected to do and can expect others to do, and reduces their control over situations (Welch and McCarville 2003). Clare can see that instead of wondering why people may resist changing the way they work, it might be more realistic to ask why they would want to accept it (Price 2008). She is not planning to change a particular aspect of practice, but to explore whether her team can alter the ethos within which they practise. Nonetheless, Clare thinks that some of the principles of managing change, particularly those concerned with the people aspects of change, may be useful in helping her to encourage people to participate in developing person-centred care. Clare expects that she will be the person leading the overall process of developing person-centred practice, and now wants to think about the best way to approach this.

Case scenario

Wajeed is part of a working group who hope to lead the development of a more person-centred approach to care on their ward. They intend to use the principles of practice development methodology to enable people to challenge the way they currently work by using reflective discussions and high challenge/high support facilitation. While they think there will be support for this in principle, they also believe that some people may not be completely behind the initiative.

*How do Wajeed and his colleagues plan to use the empirical rational, norma-
tive re-educative and power coercive approaches to change to introduce the
idea of working in a more person-centred way?*

Wajeed and his colleagues think it will be important to explain why they
are suggesting a more person-centred approach to working. This will include
what has given them this idea and why they think it is worth trying. They
believe it will be important to focus on how this will build on what the
team does well, rather than on deficits in care, so as to encourage people to
regard this as an opportunity to develop existing good practice further, not
a criticism of their current work. Wajeed also thinks that people will want to
know the practicalities of what they are being asked to do and what it will
involve. This will include how the processes of reflection will work, what
will be expected of those who participate, and how long reflective sessions
are expected to last.

The group that Wajeed is working with anticipate using the normative
re-educative approach as the mainstay of how they try to engage people with
the idea of developing person-centred care. Part of this will be to encourage
individuals and the team as a whole to own and control the way things are
developed. This will include encouraging people to explore their views on
person-centred practice, and using reflective discussions to enable people to
develop and act on their own ideas about how practice might become more
person centred. It will also involve considering issues such as the losses people
may feel, and the threats as well as opportunities that person-centred care may
bring for individuals and the team as a whole.

Wajeed and his colleagues do not intend to use the power coercive
approach, as they think it would be contrary to the principles of person-
centred care. However, they are aware that there is currently a strong emphasis
on the need to provide person-centred care throughout the hospital. Thus,
practitioners may feel that their current practice is being criticized or they are
being required to work in this way. Wajeed thinks that they should acknowledge this, but also emphasize that they see this as a way to develop what is
good in the team's work, rather than to remedy deficiencies in care.

*What losses might working in a more person-centred way bring for people in
Wajeed's team?*

Wajeed thinks that the idea of developing a more person-centred approach to
care could reduce his colleagues' security and confidence in how they work.
The way they manage their workloads may become less predictable and they
may feel that established routines are under threat. Exactly what will happen
if they move to a more person-centred approach is unknown, which is likely
to make people feel less secure about their work.

On an individual level, Wajeed knows that one nurse on his ward is seen as particularly good at coaxing patients who are reluctant to take medication or comply with other aspects of care. If a more person-centred approach is used, with a greater recognition of the individual's views, beliefs, values and perceptions making people less likely to be seen to need coaxing, this unofficial role may be lost.

Wajeed believes that the ward team currently do a very good job on a busy, demanding ward, and that being asked to explore a new approach to working could be perceived as devaluing their efforts and the quality of their work. Because of this, he wants to emphasize that developing person-centred care is intended to build on what the team do well in order to develop even better care.

What good things about current practice in Wajeed's workplace will he be able to incorporate into an ongoing narrative of person-centred care?

As well as providing good physical care, Wajeed and his colleagues try to provide patients with as much continuity of care as possible. As such, they already try to get to know patients and their relatives, and see the importance of this. They also tend to show an interest in one another and work well with other team members. Wajeed feels that as a team, they are generally committed to the 'people' aspects of care.

What aspects of working in a more person-centred way may cause Wajeed's colleagues concern?

Not having, or not perceiving themselves to have, the time to engage in reflective activities or discussions about their work is likely to be a concern for Wajeed's colleagues. There is a possibility that the practicalities of working in a more person-centred way will also be considered too time-consuming to do, even if it seems a good idea.

Wajeed's colleagues may also feel concerned about what will happen if aspects of care get missed through using a more person-centred approach. Wajeed therefore thinks that despite wanting to use a bottom-up approach to introducing person-centred care, it will be important to be seen to have managerial support for the initiative.

In addition, Wajeed thinks that people may feel uncomfortable about engaging in reflection and that the high challenge/high support approach could sound intimidating. He hopes that by identifying who will be facilitating these processes, and giving examples of how they will work, these concerns may be reduced. He also believes it will be important to emphasize that there is no one right way of being person centred, or a required outcome: it is a process.

Finally, it is possible that Wajeed's team will be concerned about how other multidisciplinary team members will view a more person-centred way of working. This may be a valid concern, as one consultant in particular has not yet accepted that the person in charge of the ward on each shift expects him to refer to different nurses to hear about different patients. Wajeed thinks that it will be important to acknowledge this potential challenge, but also to emphasize that this consultant's views have not deterred them so far and they have managerial backing for the initiative.

What will be likely to drive or restrain developing a more person-centred way of working in Wajeed's team?

Wajeed considers that the forces driving change will be that most staff on the ward genuinely want to provide good care and are interested in the people they work with. This will predispose them to becoming more person centred in their work. He also thinks that encouraging staff to participate in planning and shaping how things are done will further increase this driving force. Knowing that their managers support this approach to working is also likely to be a driving force, provided it is seen as support for the ward team's ideas, not an imposed requirement.

The restraining forces will include:

- the time required to develop person-centred processes
- the losses people may feel
- the priority people give to developing person-centred care
- the practicalities of people with busy shifts and many part-time staff getting to meetings.

Wajeed also thinks that not everyone will be enthusiastic about the idea, and the strength of the restraining force will be affected by which people resist the idea, and how much they influence others.

Who are the key opinion leaders and stakeholders on Wajeed's ward?

The key opinion leaders on Wajeed's ward are an influential group of three staff. Wajeed thinks that at least one of them is likely to be less than enthusiastic about plans to develop a more person-centred way of working. Because of their known influence, he wants one of them to be asked to join the existing working group. One of the group is relatively senior, but the other two are not. Wajeed wants to invite the one who has most influence, despite her not being the most senior, and the one most likely to oppose the idea. He hopes that by being involved, she may become more enthusiastic than Wajeed expects. If not, then the working group will at least know what likely opposition to more person-centred care they are facing and will be able to gauge the level of influence it will probably have on the rest of the ward team.

What practical resources will Wajeed's team need to develop person-centred care?

Wajeed's team will need time, a location for meetings, and someone to facilitate the process of reflecting and becoming reflexive.

Additional resources

www.changemodel.nhs.uk/pg/dashboard
Outlines the NHS change model.

www.institute.nhs.uk/quality_and_service_improvement_tools/quality_and_
service_improvement_tools/resistance_-_understanding_it.html
NHS quality and service improvement resource about resistance to change.

www.institute.nhs.uk/quality_and_service_improvement_tools/quality_and_service_
improvement_tools/human_dimensions_-_human_barriers_to_change.html
NHS quality and service improvement resource about human barriers to change.

8 Leadership and Practice Development

Chapter overview

- Successfully leading the development of person-centred practice requires a person-centred leadership style.
- Approaches that are congruent with the ethos of person-centred practice development include transformational and authentic leadership. These focus on working with people in a way that makes them want to change how they work because of the intrinsic value of doing so, not the tangible rewards that will be accrued because of it.
- Those who lead practice development initiatives may require preparation for this role and support during their work.

Carly thinks the care provided on the surgical ward where she works could be more person centred. She has discussed her thoughts with a few colleagues and the ward manager and has now been asked to take a lead on developing practice to take things in this direction. Carly would like to do this as it is something she feels strongly about, but is slightly concerned that she does not hold a senior enough position in the ward team to take the role on. She also thinks that if she does take on a leadership role in this initiative, she will need some preparation for it. So, before making a decision, she has been reading about leadership.

Leaders and managers in practice development

Carly has discovered that leadership and management are very different things and that she could take the lead in a practice development initiative without having any managerial role within her team. Management tends to be concerned with the practicalities of keeping things running smoothly within an organizational remit, including planning, budgeting and staffing. Leadership is more concerned with having a vision of how things should be and then motivating and inspiring others to follow the direction of that vision (Sheehan and Hayles 2006). It is the individual's qualities, interactions with others and ability to inspire and motivate people to share their vision that makes them a leader, not their job title or level of seniority (White 2005, Doody and Doody 2012). A manager may hold leadership qualities and be a good leader, and a leader may have management skills and responsibilities. Equally, a successful leader may not be a good manager and vice versa (Sheehan and Hayles 2006). Carly can identify from her current job and previous positions that it is not always the ward manager's ideas that people follow. It is usually someone's suggestions, and how they present them, that inspires people. She can also recall instances where the ideas that really enthused people were directly opposed to what the manager in question wanted to happen. This means that while she is not a manager, she can perhaps still lead in developing person-centred practice, if she can inspire and motivate people to want to work in a more person-centred way. Carly is committed to this way of working and has apparently also convinced the ward manager and a couple of other people that it is worth considering. She therefore thinks perhaps she can take on a leadership role in this initiative.

Practice development methodology focuses on change that is initiated and led by frontline staff, rather than that which is imposed from a managerial level (Manley and McCormack 2003). Carly thinks this further corroborates the idea that the leadership of person-centred practice need not rest with a manager. Nonetheless, having managerial support for practice development initiatives is important (McCormack et al. 2007). For person-centred care to flourish, organizations as a whole need to buy into this ethos, seek to treat others and view themselves as people, which requires managerial buy-in. In addition, the resources needed to develop practice may be hard to come by without managerial backing. This makes it important for leaders and managers to be able to work together towards a common goal of developing and sustaining person-centred cultures, despite often fulfilling different roles.

It is therefore useful if leaders can understand managerial perspectives, particularly those relating to person-centred practice development. Leaders may, for example, have a long-term vision for how things should be, but managers will often have many competing shorter term operational goals, requirements and demands, which have to be met (Carracide and Round 2004, Miller and Desmarais 2007). Leaders who understand these demands will be best placed to engage in cooperative dialogue with managers about the value of approaches such as practice development methodology, which are not designed to produce the quick or measurable changes that organizations often require (Carradice and Round 2004). By working together, leaders and managers may be able to explore how the required goals can be achieved without detracting from the central ethos of developing person-centred care. Carly has found her ward manager supportive of her thoughts and plans. However, she is also aware that as other competing organizational demands come along, she, as a leader, will need to be cognizant of these and aware of what might influence her manager's ongoing support for the development of person-centred care. Awareness of the demands placed on others also fits practice development methodology's underpinnings of critical realism and critical social theory. These acknowledge that people have differing perceptions and priorities, which need to be respected and worked with in developing person-centred cultures (Freeman and Vasconcelos 2010, Cruickshank 2012, Oliver 2012). If Carly and her ward manager can work collaboratively on developing person-centred care, it will also mean there is no conflict for other staff over whose priorities they should try to address (Boomer and McCormack 2010).

Having identified that not being in a managerial position is not necessarily a problem, but that it will be beneficial to collaborate closely with her manager, Carly is now considering whether she thinks she can be an effective leader. Leadership can be considered in two parts: one to do with vision, direction, values and purposes, and the other to do with inspiring and motivating people to work together for a common purpose (Sheehan and Hayles 2006). In terms of vision and values, Carly has a vision for person-centred care, her personal values match this, and she is highly motivated to achieve it. However, she is less confident that she can motivate other people to work together for this common purpose. So, she has decided to find out more about the different ways that leaders work to inspire and motivate people, to see if it is likely that she can achieve this.

Practice pointer 8.1

- Leadership and management are different roles and require different skills and aptitudes.
- Person-centred care will develop most effectively where leaders and managers work together to enable this to happen.

Activity 8.1

Who are the leaders in your workplace? Who are the managers?

There are many different styles of leadership, and no one approach is inherently superior or best in all situations (Sheehan and Hayles 2006). Carly intends to use practice development methodology as a way of moving towards a more person-centred approach to care, and believes that her approach to leadership should match this ethos (Bray et al. 2009, Kirkley et al. 2011, Manley et al. 2011). She has read about transactional and transformational leadership, and considered how consistent these are with practice development methodology. Transactional leadership seems to her to focus on getting people to comply with an innovation by means of material motivation and rewards. Transformational leadership, on the other hand, focuses on change being achieved because people are inspired to see things differently and thus perceive a need for change (Scott et al. 2003). The latter approach appears to Carly more congruent with practice development methodology, where people reflect on, see a need for, and an intrinsic value in, altering the way they work, rather than material incentives or rewards motivating them (Dewing 2010, Walsh et al. 2011).

Activity 8.2

Think about leaders you have worked with or observed in the past. Did any of them use a transactional approach? If so, how effective was this?

Practice pointer 8.2

- Transactional leadership focuses on achieving change by means of material motivation and rewards.
- Transformational leadership focuses on inspiring people to see things differently and thus want to change how they work.

Transformational leadership

Transformational leadership is concerned with transforming individuals and cultures. Doody and Doody (2012) describe how transformational leaders motivate people by appealing to them on the basis of morals, beliefs or values, and by engaging them emotionally and intellectually in wanting to alter the way things are. The rewards it offers are not material, but those derived from people satisfying their higher needs (Surakka 2008). This approach seems to Carly to be consistent with practice development methodology, as she wants to motivate her colleagues by promoting the intrinsic value of person-centred care and creating a shared sense of its importance (McCormack and McCance 2010). She thinks that using threats or material rewards would be inappropriate, not only because this does not match her beliefs about the best way to motivate people to change, but because person-centred working requires people to understand and value this, for its own sake. A nurse cannot, for instance, be required to genuinely engage with a patient because they will be penalized if they do not. They could be coerced in this way to carry out particular tasks, be seen to engage with people in a courteous manner, or to adjust particular aspects of the care they deliver. However, engaging in creating person-centred interactions and situations can only be achieved if the individuals and groups concerned see this as desirable, and aspire to work in this way because of its inherent value.

Transformational leaders do not need to hold positions of official authority because they do not motivate people by having the means to require them to do something. Rather, they inspire people to want to act in a particular way, regardless of who is watching or the draw of extrinsic rewards or punishments. This further encourages Carly to believe that her lack of managerial authority should not, of itself, be a barrier to her leading the development of person-centred practice.

Activity 8.3

Consider people you see, or have seen, as leaders. Did they adopt a transformational approach? If so, how effective was this?

Practice pointer 8.3

Transformational leaders motivate people by:

- appealing to them on the basis of morals, beliefs or values
- engaging them emotionally and intellectually
- the reward of doing things they see as right
- empowering people to act in a way they see as right.

They lead by inspiring, not requiring, people to work in a different way.

The approach transformational leaders adopt to achieve these outcomes is described as 'facilitative' and 'enabling' (McCormack and McCance 2010). This has resonance with practice development methodology in that, as Chapter 4 discussed, this too focuses on the processes of facilitation and enabling. Rather than giving instructions, transformational leaders enable others to reflect on and explore their own experiences and those of others, and facilitate critical dialogue that inspires people to see things differently and act in accordance with this. Carly's key role as a transformational leader would be to enable people to reflect on and explore their experiences and creatively consider the possibility of more person-centred ways of working (McCormack and McCance 2010). Ideas about how practice should develop would not come from Carly; instead, she would lead a process by which other team members generated the ideas that brought about transformations in their thinking and working (McCormack and McCance 2010). Carly can see that this links with the bottom-up approach to change seen in practice development methodology, where frontline workers develop and act on ideas about what should change and why.

The principles of transformational leadership therefore seem to Carly to be consistent with practice development methodology, and an approach that would work for promoting more person-centred care. To achieve change using this approach, she, as a leader, would need to inspire and motivate others to see the ideal of person-centred care as important enough to act on (Doody and Doody 2012). This means that she would need to speak, but also act, in a way that inspired and motivated others to view more person-centred care as desirable, to aspire to work in this way, and see it as achievable (McCormack and McCance 2010). Her actions would include her interactions with patients, but also with her colleagues, and whether or not she was seen to be reflective and reflexive in her own practice, as discussed in Chapter 4 (Boomer and McCormack 2010).

Carly thinks that using a transformational approach would be a good way of leading the development of more person-centred practice in her workplace. However, she is not sure she can be the charismatic and inspiring leader that it requires. She has also came across the concept of authentic leadership, which seems consistent with practice development methodology and which she thinks she could work with more confidently.

Authentic leadership

A core value of person-centredness is authenticity, where individuals interact openly and honestly, as people, with one another (Sanders et al. 2013). Authentic leadership appears to Carly to have logical links with the ethos of person-centred practice development (Branson 2007). In addition, like transformational leadership, it is focused on inspiring people to want to take actions that fit a particular value system, rather than coercing them to do things because of the consequences of not doing so (Branson 2007).

Authentic leadership has four central attributes: self-awareness, balanced processing, moral self-identity, and relational transparency. However, the key attribute that underpins all the others is self-awareness (Branson 2007, Diddams and Chang 2012). Authentic leaders, like transformational leaders, have clarity about their values and convictions, but their actions are closely guided by self-knowledge. This means they understand their own ideals, strengths, weaknesses, what is likely to influence their thoughts, perceptions and the way in which they make sense of the world (Branson 2007, Avolio et al. 2009, Diddimas and Chang 2012). An authentic leader understands their inner self, motives, values and beliefs, and uses this self-knowledge to interpret their reality and become more aware of the tacit truths that govern what they choose to do (Branson 2007). This self-knowledge means they have integrity in their decision making and actions (Diddams and Chang 2012). Authentic leadership therefore involves more than knowing what one is or wishes to be, and includes an understanding of what drives this and the ability to question one's motivations and motives. Carly thinks this has clear links to the focus in practice development methodology on becoming and being reflective and reflexive, and aware of oneself and what motivates one (Peek et al. 2007, Dewing 2010, Brown and McCormack 2011).

Practice pointer 8.4

The attributes of authentic leadership are:

- self-awareness
- balanced processing
- moral self-identity
- relational transparency.

Authentic leaders take into account the interplay between one individual's actions and the lives and actions of others (Diddams and Chang 2012). As well as being aware of their own inner beings, they are aware of how others perceive their thinking and behaviour, and how the context in which they operate influences how their actions are viewed (Avolio et al. 2009). This seems to Carly to relate to what she has read about the critical realism and critical social theory that are influential in practice development methodology, where the individual cannot be separated from their context and social milieu (Freeman and Vasconcelos 2010, Bevan et al. 2012, Cruickshank 2012, Lapum et al. 2012, Oliver 2012).

Developing this type of self-knowledge requires ongoing and deliberate effort by the person concerned, through feedback from others but also reflective self-inquiry and self-evaluation (Branson 2007, Sanders et al. 2013). This key element of authentic leadership appears to Carly to have a natural fit with the ongoing reflective processes seen in practice development methodology, and to be consistent with leading a person-centred practice development initiative.

Practice pointer 8.5

With regard to self-awareness and authentic leadership, authentic leaders:

* understand their own ideals, strengths and weaknesses
* are aware of what influences their thoughts and perceptions
* can question their own motives
* perceive the interplay between one individual's actions and the lives and actions of others
* consider how their thinking and behaviour is perceived by others
* are aware of how the context in which they operate influences their actions and how these are perceived.

Balanced processing is the second element of authentic leadership. This concerns the leader being able to objectively analyse relevant information before making a decision (Avolio et al. 2009, Walumbwa et al. 2010, Diddams and Chang 2012). It includes them actively seeking input from others and non-defensively considering this. Carly thinks this is consistent with the ethos of shared decision making seen as crucial to person-centred practice (McCormack et al. 2010, Manley et al. 2011, McKay et al. 2012, van den Pol-Grevelink et al. 2012). It is also congruent with critical realism's acknowledgement of the importance of different types of knowledge and perspectives in understanding people and situations (Oliver 2012).

While balanced processing seeks to objectively analyse information, it does not presume perfect objectivity; rather, it means that a leader is able to collect and process the information they are presented with without threat to their own ego (Gardner et al. 2005). Their objectivity may be limited, encompassing the acknowledgement seen in critical realism that complete objectivity is often elusive (Oliver 2012), but their interpretation of reality is not constrained by defensiveness on their part. Authentic leaders have the ability to see things from different angles and are able to take into consideration different needs and perceptions, without reacting in a negative or defensive manner (May et al. 2003).

Practice pointer 8.6

With regard to balanced processing and authentic leadership, authentic leaders:

* actively seek input from others
* can see things from different angles
* consider different people's needs and perceptions
* collect and process the information they are presented with without feeling threatened or reacting negatively.

A third attribute of authentic leadership is moral self-identity, which refers to the leader's ability to be guided by internal moral standards and use these to regulate their behaviour (Avolio et al. 2009, Walumbwa et al. 2010, Diddams and Chang 2012). This is similar to the moral underpinnings of transformational leadership, but in authentic leaders it is combined with a self-awareness, which means that the leader understands why they hold the moral standpoint they do, and have questioned, and continue to question, this. Thus, an authentic leader has moral fortitude or resilience: they can act in a way that matches their beliefs and values and are able to sustain such actions despite setbacks or pressure to do otherwise (Avolio et al. 2009).

Practice pointer 8.7

With regard to moral self-identity and authentic leadership, authentic leaders:

- are guided by internal moral standards
- understand why they hold the moral standpoint they do
- continue to act according to their moral standards despite pressure to do otherwise.

The final attribute of authentic leadership is relational transparency, meaning that leaders act transparently and openly with others. Without feeling threatened or needing to adopt defensive or coercive behaviour, their self-awareness and moral self-identity enable them to explain and explore why they see things as they do and make the recommendations they make (Diddams and Chang 2012). This sharing is, however, focused on what is authentic and appropriate to the situation in question. For instance, while sharing feelings, beliefs and perceptions is likely to be appropriate, coercive displays of emotion are not (Avolio et al. 2009).

Practice pointer 8.8

With regard to relational transparency and authentic leadership, authentic leaders:

- act transparently and openly with others
- can explain and explore why they see things as they do.

Carly sees many of the attributes of authentic leaders as similar to those of transformational leaders but notes a distinction, in that authentic leaders are not necessarily charismatic (Diddams and Chang 2012). They do not primarily motivate others by inspirational vision or intellectual stimulation. Instead, they promote trust because their deep self-knowledge creates a non-defensiveness that allows them to be consistent in their behaviours and dialogues, and transparent about the reasons for their actions (Wong and Cummings, 2009). This appeals to Carly because she thinks that while she may not be able to be a charismatic or transformational leader, she can work on developing her ability to be an authentic leader. She also thinks this will be compatible with what she and her colleagues need to achieve in terms of developing person-centred practice.

Activity 8.4

Think about leaders you have worked with or seen. Did they use an authentic approach in terms of:

- self-awareness
- balanced processing
- moral self-identity
- relational transparency?

How effective were they in engaging people to follow them?

Nonetheless, authentic leadership presents some challenges. Truthful self-awareness is the cornerstone of authentic leadership, but the development of self-awareness includes acknowledgment of one's weaknesses, ambiguities, inconsistencies and limitations in self-knowledge (Diddams and Chang 2012). This is a key aspect of authentic leadership, in that a part of the trust people develop for their leaders arises from their ability to appropriately acknowledge their limitations as well as strengths. However, as leaders become aware of their own weaknesses, they may become less willing to disclose the totality of who they are to their followers for fear that their limitations will be off-putting (Diddams and Chang 2012). Carly wants, in theory, to have the confidence to be an authentic leader, who can recognize and acknowledge her weaknesses as well as strengths, but can see that she will probably need support in developing and sustaining this ability.

An authentic leader not only develops self-awareness, but also constantly reviews and interprets their own beliefs and values. Their self-awareness is not, therefore, static (Diddams and Chang 2012). While this is a necessary part of being authentic, it can become problematic as leaders will, almost inevitably, realize that they have perceived things, including themselves, in a mistaken way in the past (Nussbaum and Dweck, 2008). Because one can only be authentic in terms of one's current level of self-knowledge, there may be some apparent ambiguity in a person's authenticity as their awareness changes. The relational transparency seen in authentic leadership is important in this respect as it enables leaders to explain and be open about how changes in their perceptions, including their perceptions of themselves, influence their views and actions over time.

Authentic leadership requires development and sustenance. This can be achieved through the processes of facilitation aimed at enabling leaders to develop, maintain and deepen their authenticity, and accept the changes in their perspectives and self-knowledge this will bring (Sanders et al. 2013). Carly would like to use the principles of authentic leadership, but recognizes that she needs to prepare herself for this and its challenges. In addition, she wants to gain skills and confidence in some of the practicalities of leadership with which she is not familiar. In her quest for ways in which she may be able to develop her leadership skills and knowledge, she has come across the ACES model.

ACES model

The ACES model represents four distinct, but interrelated domains of leadership development: the analytical (A), conceptual (C), emotional (E) and spiritual (S) domains (Quatro et al. 2007).

Practice pointer 8.9

The ACES model (Quatro et al. 2007) comprises four interrelated but distinct domains of leadership development: analytical, conceptual, emotional and spiritual.

Analytical domain

The analytical domain concerns developing leaders who can understand and manage complexity. It includes practical skills in planning, organizing, problem solving, monitoring performance and trends, and clarifying roles and objectives, but also stresses the cognitive abilities underpinning these processes. For example, problem solving requires the information that is available from a range of sources to be processed in a systematic manner so as to identify the causes of problems as well as potential solutions. Carly thinks this will be useful for her, because although she aims to use a leadership approach that focuses on developing reflective self-knowledge, she knows that practical and organizational skills and abilities will also be valuable assets.

In addition, this domain includes the concept of leaders giving feedback, which is an area Carly thinks she will need to develop. While she will not be taking on a managerial role, she believes that leading the development of person-centred practice will require her to have the ability to provide effective feedback on the person-centredness of the care she sees people delivering.

She is aware of the importance of feedback being timely, regular and relevant, and focusing on good quality care and people's strengths, as well as areas that could be improved (Donnelly and Kirk 2010, Busser 2012). She also recognizes that effective feedback requires those giving and those receiving feedback to feel listened to, understood and respected. This necessitates the use of open-ended questions, and for the person providing feedback to listen to the other person's perspectives in order to facilitate a two-way dialogue about perceptions, interpretations of situations and rationales for actions (Busser 2012). However, despite having some understanding of the principles of giving effective feedback, Carly thinks she needs to build on this and develop practical skills, as well as theoretical knowledge, in this area.

Looking at this part of the ACES model has highlighted skills Carly thinks she could usefully seek opportunities to develop.

Practice pointer 8.10

The analytical domain of the ACES model (Quatro et al. 2007) concerns developing leaders who:

- can understand and manage complexity
- possess practical skills in planning, organizing, problem solving and monitoring
- have the cognitive abilities to underpin these processes.

Conceptual domain

The conceptual domain of the ACES model concerns developing leaders who can understand and manage complex, multifactorial situations and work creatively within these (Quatro et al. 2007). Like the analytical domain, it includes developing a leader's cognitive abilities and skills, but focuses more strongly on inductive reasoning and creatively synthesizing information from a range of sources. Developing these abilities enables leaders to understand complex issues and problems and develop new ways of addressing them. Carly sees links between this and practice development methodology in terms of synthesizing information of different types and from different sources, the acknowledgment of different perceptions of reality, and the importance of critical creativity (Manley et al. 2013a). The conceptual domain also includes elements she thinks will be valuable to her in developing the skills of balanced processing so that she can non-defensively consider differing viewpoints and perspectives.

The development of a strong conceptual capacity allows leaders to get at the heart of complex problems, and, by role modelling this, enables them to motivate others to explore issues in depth (Quatro et al. 2007). Carly thinks this approach has some links to the critical, in-depth reflection her team will need to engage in when using practice development methodology, and that by developing this skill herself, she will be better able to role model it to the rest of the ward team.

Practice pointer 8.11

The conceptual domain of the ACES model (Quatro et al. 2007) concerns developing leaders who:

- can understand and manage interrelated complexity
- foster creativity
- are able to use inductive as well as deductive reasoning
- can creatively synthesize information from a range of sources.

Emotional domain

The emotional domain of the ACES model concerns developing leaders who are skilled at noting, understanding and managing human emotion in themselves and others and leveraging these as a source of energy and influence (Quatro et al. 2007). Carly can relate this to what she had read about transformational leadership and the charismatic qualities of some leaders. However, it also seems important in developing the skills required of an authentic leader in terms of self-knowledge and awareness of how others respond to her. In addition, it appears to be a key element of developing relational transparency in terms of not being threatened or led to defensive behaviour by negative emotions (Quatro et al. 2007). Carly thinks that developing the emotional domain of leadership will be a key aspect of becoming an authentic leader.

Practice pointer 8.12

The emotional domain of the ACES model (Quatro et al. 2007) concerns developing leaders who:

- are skilled at noting, understanding and managing human emotion
- can use emotion in themselves and others as a source of energy and influence.

Spiritual domain

The spiritual domain of leadership focuses on leaders enabling their followers to connect individual tasks and larger goals to deeply held moral and ethical values (Quatro et al. 2007). Quatro et al. (2007) suggest that this may be especially relevant to enabling transformational leaders to progress to a stage of development in which they act in an independent and ethical manner, regardless of the expectations of individuals or the norms of society. Carly thinks it also has links with the strong moral self-identity seen in authentic leaders and will therefore be an important part of developing her skills in this type of leadership. It will assist her to motivate others to want to work in a more person-centred way, but also to develop the moral fortitude to stay focused on developing person-centred care despite challenges or setbacks.

Practice pointer 8.13

The spiritual domain of the ACES model (Quatro et al. 2007) concerns developing leaders who enable others to connect tasks and goals to moral and ethical values.

Carly likes the idea of using the ACES model to plan her own leadership development. Its four domains focus on the emotional and spiritual aspects of leadership as well as the practicalities, which she thinks will be important in trying to inspire people to want to practise is a more person-centred way. At the same time, she wants to become more adept in the practicalities of leadership, so that her theoretical ideals translate into actions.

Activity 8.5

Consider your own strengths and weaknesses as a leader in terms of the four domains of the ACES model: analytical, conceptual, emotional and spiritual. Which areas would you want to develop?

Leadership development

Carly now feels she will be able to take on a leadership role in developing person-centred practice. Nevertheless, she still thinks her skills and confidence in performing this role require development, both at the outset and throughout her leadership journey (White 2005). The reading she has done on transformational and authentic leadership has given her some ideas about how she would like to function as a leader. In addition, the ACES model has provided her with some useful pointers regarding the sort of personal and professional development and support she will need to help her develop her leadership skills. Although Carly has looked at leadership development programmes, she has decided she wants to create her own learning programme, focused on her specific needs.

A key skill Carly thinks she needs to develop and hone is the ability to be reflective and self-aware. If the ward is to move to a more person-centred approach to care, this will be a part of the practice development journey for all concerned. However, Carly wants to work on developing her own ability to reflect and be reflexive, so that as well as being a part of this process, she can lead by example. Miller and Desmarais (2007) identify the importance of mentorship programmes for leaders, and Carly thinks this would be useful for her. The principles of high challenge/high support (as described in Chapter 4) match how Carly would like a mentor to work with her (Manley et al. 2009, McCormack et al. 2009, Titchen et al. 2013). She wants to find someone who will be truthful and really challenging, but also supportive of her, as she develops her leadership skills (White 2005). Carly believes that if someone can work with her in this way, it will assist her to develop her self-knowledge, skills in balanced processing, moral conviction and resilience. To achieve this, her mentor will need to be someone whose values and way of working are congruent with what Carly is aiming for. She has identified a ward manager on another ward who she thinks would be an ideal mentor, but is mindful this would take time, from her own ward and theirs. She is also aware that she needs to be tactful in approaching her own ward manager about this idea, so that they do not feel that their own leadership and support skills are being devalued. She plans to present her idea as being linked to the value of having an outsider, who can view things with fresh eyes, to mentor her, rather than there being an absence of people who could provide this type of mentorship on her own ward.

As well as identifying who may be able to work with her in a mentorship capacity, Carly is reflecting on who, in the past, she had seen as an inspirational leader and can learn from, albeit retrospectively (Kempster 2009). She has begun to develop a reflective leadership journal in which she consciously thinks about leaders she has learned from in the past. This includes what it was she saw in them that she now seeks to emulate, how they worked and what made this effective. She is also reflecting on leaders she thinks did not work as she would want to and why this was, and is trying to link these thoughts to her own ideals and plans for leadership. They are reflections she thinks she will ultimately share in reflective discussions with a mentor, but they currently give her a starting point for developing ideas about her own approach to leadership.

In addition, Carly wants to develop her skills and confidence in the more concrete aspects of leadership, such as her decision-making and planning skills. She believes that having more confidence in these areas will help her to be more comfortable with the decisions she makes and enhance her ability to transform her ideals and plans into action. She thinks she can work on many of these things with her mentor, but is also looking for study days or master classes about particular aspects of leadership that she might want to attend.

> **Practice pointer 8.14**
>
> Leadership development may include:
>
> * accessing specific information
> * developing specific skills
> * mentorship
> * learning from current role models
> * reflecting on one's own actions
> * reflecting on the way in which past role models led.

Summary

Carly thinks that the transformational and authentic leadership styles are both congruent with practice development methodology. However, she also believes the approach to leadership she will adopt does not necessarily need to subscribe in whole to one model or approach: she can use particular aspects of specific models or approaches at different times, as appropriate (Doody and Doody 2012). The key thing for her is that the way in which she acts, as a leader, should be consistent with the principles of person-centredness. Although Carly understands that leaders need not be managers, she also sees the benefits of leaders and managers working together to achieve effective developments in practice.

While Carly is currently focusing on how she will develop her leadership skills, she is also considering the practicalities of how she will introduce the idea of developing more person-centred practice. A part of this is thinking about how she will know if her attempts to introduce a more person-centred approach to care are having a positive influence on what happens in practice.

Case scenario

Anita thinks the 10-bed burns unit where she works could adopt a more person-centred approach to care. However, she is not sure that she wants to lead the process of trying to encourage people to work in this way. Anita is considering whether to try to persuade another person that it is worth the unit trying to adopt a more person-centred approach to practice, so that they can lead the process of achieving this, or to attempt to develop her own leadership skills in order to do this herself. She has begun by thinking about who the leaders and managers in her workplace are, so that she knows who she might target to persuade to lead the process or assist her in leading it.

The leaders and managers in Anita's workplace

The manager of the burns unit is the charge nurse. Two junior sisters assist in managing the unit and deputize for him. There is also a matron who has managerial responsibility for the surgical unit as a whole, and whose jurisdiction the burns unit comes under.

The charge nurse's role is concerned with the smooth day-to-day running of the unit, ensuring that it is adequately staffed, policies and protocols are kept to, budgets are not exceeded, staff are treated fairly, standards of care are adhered to, and patients and relatives are satisfied with the care provided. He is generally thought to be a fair manager, well organized, and a clinical expert in caring for patients who have suffered burns.

The leaders on the unit include one of the junior sisters, who often convinces others to do things in the way she thinks is most appropriate. She has a degree of authority because of her position, but it tends to be her conviction about ideas and how she explains these that convinces others, not her managerial role. Another leader is one of the staff nurses who is often listened to by others, and who frequently convinces people to do, or not do, things. She does not have any official authority to enable her to achieve this, but it seems to Anita that the force of her personality and her ability to make things difficult if people do not do as she suggests encourages people to follow what she says.

Do any of the leaders on Anita's unit adopt a transactional approach? If so, how effective is this?

Anita thinks that the staff nurse referred to above influences others using a form of transactional leadership, in that there are tangible rewards or punishments for one's actions in terms of how one is regarded and spoken to by her. In addition, she often convinces people to follow what she says based on it being a more efficient way to work, or there not being time to get everything done any other way. This suggests a reward for working in the way she advocates in terms of time and effort, rather than the intrinsic reward of working in a better way.

This approach seems to Anita to be effective at times, because people tend to do things as this staff nurse wants. However, it generally only happens when she is there. In between times, her influence is minimal. Nonetheless, over time, if she convinces more and more people, more and more regularly, to work as she wants them to, things do change permanently.

Do any of the leaders on Anita's unit adopt a transformational approach? If so, how effective is this?

Anita considers that the junior sister adopts a transformational approach to leadership. She has the type of personality and enthusiasm that encourages others to come on board with her ideas, and has a way of speaking to people and explaining why things would be beneficial that makes them want to be a part of doing what she suggests. Her appeal to people is not based on any suggestion of material or tangible rewards or benefits, but by engaging them in wanting to work in a particular way. This includes people seeing how she works and wanting to emulate this.

This approach to leadership seems very effective. People appear to engage with the ideas the junior sister promotes and genuinely seek to carry them through, even when she is not there, because they see them as important. Although the junior sister could use her position to encourage others to work as she suggests, she tends not to do so. Her approach to motivating others is based on engaging with them to help them to see why what she suggests is a good idea and beneficial for patients and staff. Anita does not recall there being any adverse consequences per se from not doing as she suggests, but people tend to support her, and thus there is perhaps a degree of peer pressure from her followers that encourages others to conform.

Has Anita worked with anyone who used an authentic approach to leadership in terms of self-awareness, balanced processing, moral self-identity or relational transparency? How effective were they in engaging people to follow them?

Anita does not think the leaders on the burns unit are authentic leaders in its full form, although many of the junior sister's actions fulfil parts of authentic leadership. She shows self-awareness, knows her own ideals, strengths and weaknesses, and is guided by and able to stay with her moral standpoint. However, Anita is less certain that she actively seeks input from others and can see things from different angles. Although she does not seem to feel threatened or react badly if people disagree with her, she tends to continue to follow her own path, rather than engaging in considering the views that other people offer. She does, however, act transparently and openly with others and can explain why she sees things as she does. What Anita feels is lacking in terms of authenticity in her leadership is the ability to engage with others in exploring different perspectives on ideas and questioning herself.

Anita has compared this situation with a ward sister she worked with when she was newly qualified. This person was fairly quiet and, when people first met her, they often thought she would be easy to manipulate. However, she had strong moral and ethical principles that guided her work and meant that, even when opposed, she could remain true to her course. She was, nonetheless, ready to engage with people, explore their viewpoints and hers, how they differed, why they differed, and was prepared to change her perspective in the light of new information or understanding. She showed herself to be self-aware, but also able to acknowledge that she was still developing and refining her awareness of herself and her world. People respected her, because although she had clear principles and ideals that guided her work, she was also willing to admit to being human. She seemed to understand how others might feel and react and, even when she did not agree with them, showed respect for them and their views. Anita recalled that the ward always felt like an open and honest environment that everyone, including patients, benefitted from.

This leadership style seemed effective, because people understood what the ward sister asked them to do, why she saw it as important, and were generally convinced that she sought to act in patients' best interests. However, they were also encouraged to think about and question what they did, and what others, including the ward sister, did. The ward, as Anita recalled, worked well because there was respect for their leader, but she also respected them, and there was an unspoken expectation that they would respect one another.

Anita's strengths and weaknesses as a leader in terms of the ACES model

Analytical

Anita thinks her practical skills in planning, organizing and problem solving are quite good. However, these mostly relate to direct patient care, not leading others. She feels that she lacks knowledge and experience in monitoring performance and trends, and clarifying roles and objectives.

Conceptual

Anita considers herself to be good at managing some complex issues, such as complex patient care, but is less confident with the complexity of managing staff. She thinks that she often looks deductively, not inductively, at problems and their solutions, and while she works well in a technical sense, she is not very creative in solving problems.

Emotional

Anita believes that she is skilled at noting, understanding and managing human emotion in others. However, she is more confident in her ability to achieve this in relation to patients than to staff, is not always good at managing her own emotions, and often feels upset when people oppose what she says or criticize her. She is not good at leveraging emotions, especially negative ones, in herself or other staff, as sources of energy and influence.

Spiritual

Anita is not sure that she could enable other people to connect individual tasks and the larger goal to moral and ethical values. At present, she feels she lacks the confidence and conviction to do this.

What areas of leadership does Anita want to develop?

Anita thinks that in order to develop leadership skills, she will first need to develop her confidence in managing her own and other people's views, emotions and reactions. At present, despite thinking that developing a more person-centred approach to care would be good, she knows that if she proposes this and the suggestion does not meet with enthusiasm, she will feel unhappy and back down. She thinks that working with someone to help her become more confident in stating her views, and responding to how they are received, will be a useful starting point. To achieve this, she feels she will need a mentor or facilitator with whom she can discuss events at work and her feelings about them. She has decided to look out for any study opportunities that indicate they focus on this type of development, but also to think about who she can ask to act as a mentor or facilitator for her.

Anita recognizes that in order to lead developments in practice, she will also have to work on the spiritual aspects of her leadership capacity, and develop some of her analytical and conceptual abilities into leadership as well as patient care skills. However, she believes that working on the emotional aspects of leadership first will prepare her to enter into the spiritual elements, and assist her to be ready and confident to develop and transfer her existing analytical and conceptual skills to leadership situations.

Anita has decided she is not yet ready to lead this practice development initiative on her own. However, she feels that developing a more person-centred approach to care is important, and has therefore decided to approach the junior sister, whose leadership style she likes, to see if they can work together on it. If she agrees, Anita can use this as an opportunity to develop her leadership skills as well as working alongside someone else on developing person-centred care.

Additional resources

Authentic leadership
http://leadership.uoregon.edu/resources/exercises_tips/leadership_reflections/10_things_authentic_leaders_do
Describes 10 things authentic leaders do.

http://digitalcommons.unl.edu/cgi/viewcontent.cgi?article=1021&context=managementfacpub
A study of the qualities of authentic leadership.

Transformational leadership
http://changingminds.org/disciplines/leadership/styles/transformational_leadership.htm
www.cio.com/article/2384791/careers-staffing/how-to-apply-transformational-leadership-at-your-company.html
Describe transformational leaders and their qualities.

9 Evaluating Practice Development

Chapter overview

- Evaluating the consequences of attempts to develop person-centred practice is a key part of practice development methodology.
- The evaluation of person-centred practice development should explore the perspectives of all those concerned and meaningfully involve all key stakeholders.
- Realistic evaluation may be useful in evaluating person-centred practice development, because it integrates different types of knowledge and places events in their social and contextual situation.
- Designing an evaluation requires consideration of what will be evaluated, how it will be evaluated, who will collect evaluative information, how this information will be analysed, and the ethical issues associated with evaluative processes.

David is one of the senior registered nurses in a residential home for older people. Over the past six months, he has been using the principles of practice development methodology to lead the process of trying to develop more person-centred care in his workplace. The reflective discussions the team have been involved in indicate that people now generally intend to work in a more person-centred way and David thinks this intention is borne out in practice. However, he wants to evaluate whether this is truly the case and if the process of using practice development methodology has improved things for anyone. He would also like to know what has made the process of developing person-centred practice work, or detracted from its success (Cork 2005, Welford 2006, Reid et al. 2007). David is now exploring how he can conduct the evaluation in a way that matches the ethos of person-centred practice development.

> **Practice pointer 9.1**
>
> The way developments in practice are evaluated should be congruent with the ethos underpinning them. Person-centred practice development should be evaluated using approaches that match this ethos.

Person-centred evaluation

David wants to use an approach to evaluation that is consistent with the person-centred ethos he has been striving to develop in his workplace. This means it being inclusive of all those involved and enabling them to participate as equal partners in the evaluation process (McCormack et al. 2013). As Chapter 5 identified, patients should be key players in any practice development initiative, and David has worked with a small group that includes representatives of residents, their families and staff in developing person-centred practice. He considers it important for this partnership working with residents and relatives to continue during the evaluation process.

As well as being person centred, David wants the evaluation to reflect the principles of critical social theory and critical realism that underpin practice development methodology (Freeman and Vasconcelos 2010, Bevan et al. 2012, Lapum et al. 2012, Oliver 2012, Parlour and McCormack 2012). This means that the approach used has to cater for the complex personally, contextually and socially constructed nature of reality, and acknowledge that there is no one universally perceived or accepted 'truth'. However, it will still need to provide a faithful representation of what constitutes the reality or realities of the situation in the home. If the evaluation does not achieve this, then practice that directly affects residents and staff will be influenced by inaccurate information. David's evaluation will therefore need to be rigorous and systematic, although it will not aim to identify single, generalizable truths, facts, causes or effects (Manley et al. 2011).

An approach David has come across whose principles he thinks closely match what he wants to achieve is realistic evaluation.

> **Practice pointer 9.2**
>
> Practice development methodology acknowledges the complex personal, contextual and socially constructed nature of reality, and that many different truths exist, in different circumstances. The evaluation of person-centred practice development activities should be consistent with this acknowledgment.

Realistic evaluation

David is interested in finding out what is, and is not, working well in the process of developing person-centred care in his workplace. He is not concerned about the generalizability of what he finds, as he does not intend to apply it to anywhere other than the home he works in. So, he wants to use an approach that focuses on acknowledging and exploring, rather than trying to minimize, the contextual factors that contribute to whether or not person-centred care is being achieved. Realistic evaluation, like practice development methodology, is strongly influenced by the belief that people and their social context are critical factors in the success or otherwise of any intervention (Timmins and Miller 2007). It aims to identify what works in different contexts and why it works, but does not claim generalizability (Tolson and Schofield 2012).

Practice pointer 9.3

The processes used to evaluate person-centred practice development should be rigorous and systematic and provide a true representation of the realities and perceptions of reality that exist.

Realistic evaluation also seems to David to match the person-centred focus of practice development methodology, as it looks at events from the perspectives of all key stakeholders – in this case, residents, families and staff (Pittam et al. 2010). In addition, while it focuses on the people involved, and their perspectives and perceptions, realistic evaluation seeks to use these different perspectives to explain why things happen as they do, or are perceived as they are (Holma and Kontinen 2011). David considers this important, as he does not just want to understand what individuals feel and do, but why this is the case.

Activity 9.1

If you were evaluating developments in person-centred care in your workplace, whose experiences and perspectives would you need to explore?

Like critical realism, realistic evaluation acknowledges the complex functioning of the social world (Holma and Kontinen 2011, Parlour and McCormack 2012, Porter and O'Halloran 2012). It recognizes the importance of context and circumstances on the success or otherwise of interventions, but also that perceptions and constructions of reality can change over time

(McGaughey et al. 2010, Wand et al. 2011). In realistic evaluation, outcomes are linked to the social and cultural conditions they occur in and when they occur (Rycroft-Malone et al. 2009). For example, whether people in David's team feel able to practise in a person-centred way may vary from day to day depending on who they are working with, how they feel, what else is happening, what other people say to them, how much time they have and suchlike. Realistic evaluation does not look for strict correlations between single events, but instead seeks to explain how different phenomena are associated with one another in particular circumstances, and therefore what works, when, for whom and why (Jeyasingham 2008, Rycroft-Malone et al. 2010, Holma and Kontinen 2011). David thinks this will be important in his evaluation, because the nuances of each day may make a significant difference to how people feel about providing person-centred care, and how person centred the care they provide is.

Practice development methodology and realistic evaluation both embrace the concept of using different types of knowledge, including experiential, intuitive and tacit knowledge, as well as measurable, observable information (Lhussier et al. 2008). This appeals to David, because many of the changes in care provision he has seen and heard about in reflective groups concern small, immeasurable, but significant everyday encounters. The reflective discussions he has been engaged in also suggest it is this type of knowledge that often influences people's perceptions and actions.

Practice pointer 9.4

Realistic evaluation:

- investigates the perspectives of all key stakeholders
- sees the social context of events as important
- recognizes that perceptions may change according to time and context
- explores why things happen or are perceived as they are
- uses different types of knowledge to gain in-depth understanding.

Realistic evaluation distinguishes between a theory being problematic, and the way it is implemented being problematic (Pedersen et al. 2012). For instance, it would include whether person-centred care was, in principle, a good idea, and whether people wanted to achieve it, but also whether they practised in this way, in what circumstances they found this possible or impossible and why this was. It also assumes that a particular intervention is not the only thing occurring at a given time. Instead, it looks to identify all the things that are happening and how they interact with and influence each other (Porter and O'Halloran 2012). Realistic evaluation would see it as important to explore how the process of person-centred care being introduced has affected its implementation. It would also consider it necessary to look at how any other changes in the workplace and demands being placed on David's colleagues have influenced whether or not staff feel able to practise in this way.

Having read about realistic evaluation, David thinks it will be a useful framework for him to use to structure the evaluation of person-centred care in his workplace. However, he has also considered its origins to see if it will be directly transferable to his setting. As described by Pawson and Tilley (1997), realistic evaluation deals with developing a theory, and then testing this theory in terms of the context (C) in which it occurs, the mechanisms (M) used to implement the theory, and the outcomes (O) of these mechanisms being put into place – the CMO process. The origins of realistic evaluation concerned theories and mechanisms that were fairly easily defined, such as a theory about whether placing CCTV cameras in particular locations would reduce crime, and outcomes that were more tangible than those related to person-centred approaches to care (Timmins and Miller 2007). However, David thinks that, despite liking the principles of realistic evaluation, he will probably need to adapt these slightly in order to use them to evaluate person-centred care. He has, for instance, found that other evaluators who used this approach for less concrete interventions encountered difficulties in identifying and defining the exact contexts, mechanisms and outcomes involved (Timmins and Miller 2007). As a result, he has tried to determine the theory, context and mechanisms he is exploring, and the outcomes he is interested in, so as to identify how far these can be linked to the CMO process of realistic evaluation.

Realistic evaluation begins with a theory about what will work and in what circumstances it will work (Pawson and Tilley 1997, Tolson and Schofield 2012). David has decided that he does not have a theory, but instead has a question he wants to answer. This question is whether, as a result of using the principles of practice development methodology, his team has begun to work in a more person-centred way.

Contexts are the settings within which the theory being evaluated is located. This includes not just the physical context, but also the history and structures of the organization, people's priorities and motivations, and the organizational culture. In David's case, the context is a 20-bed residential home for older people, with 42 staff, many of whom work part time and most of whom are care assistants. The home is privately owned. The owner visits quite frequently and is keen on the idea of trying to move to a more person-centred approach to care. All staff have regular updates on mandatory elements of care, but few engage in any other continuous professional development. Those who live at the home are often in residential care because they have become too physically frail to cope at home. A few suffer with dementia, although those with advanced disease cannot currently be catered for. Many residents have families who visit regularly. The home has a large sitting area, which was, until recently, arranged with chairs round the edge and a large TV in one corner. Residents are encouraged to use the sitting room during the day and various activities are organized there. The home has a small garden the residents can use, and group outings away from the home are occasionally organized for them.

Before the current attempt to move to a more person-centred approach to care, David thought the care provided was somewhat ritualistic. Although he had never considered there to be any unkindness to or maltreatment of residents, he had begun to feel that perhaps the respect they deserved as people was a little lacking. Staff seemed to feel that as they were busy, doing things in rather a ritualistic way was the only way to get through the day's tasks. The culture of the home appeared to be that the priority was to get through the necessary tasks. At the time when person-centred care was being considered, a refurbishment of the home was also being planned, and the owner was looking into taking people with greater care needs, including those with advanced dementia and Alzheimer's disease.

Activity 9.2

How would you describe the context of your workplace?

Mechanisms are the things people do to produce the desired outcomes. David thinks the mechanisms in this case are the tools of practice development methodology, as described in Chapter 4. These include working in partnership with residents and families in the process of developing practice, individual and group reflection, and critical companionship.

The outcome of interest to David is whether care is now more person centred, why this is, and how the various aspects of the context and mechanisms have combined to make the outcome what it is. This is unlikely to be a measurable outcome, because it will concern how the key stakeholders involved view the way in which care is now provided.

The process of realistic evaluation is intended to test and then allow refining and retesting of the original theory (Rycroft-Malone et al. 2011, Jackson and Kolla 2012). In addition, because it focuses heavily on context, realistic evaluation acknowledges that something that works at one point in time cannot be assumed to work forever, or in all circumstances (Rycroft-Malone et al. 2009). In this respect, it has links with the cyclical nature of action research, as described in Chapter 6, which is often used in practice development methodology. David intends this evaluation to be a part of a process of ongoing development and evaluation of person-centred practice. He is also aware that as staff come and go and residents and families change, things at the home may alter because of the different people involved and how they interact to create the culture of the home. Thus, ongoing cycles of evaluation and action will be important if person-centred practice is to continue to be developed and refined.

Having considered the principles and origin of realistic evaluation and what his modified CMO might be, David thinks he can use these principles in his evaluation of person-centred care. His next step is to decide, in practical terms, what he will evaluate and how he will achieve this.

What to evaluate

Evaluation generally includes determining whether or not something has happened, the process by which this happened, and its effect (Reid et al. 2007). David will be evaluating whether or not care has become more person centred, thus he needs to define what this means and what he expects the outcome of more person-centred care to be. He has found this slightly challenging, because what person-centred care means and what it looks like are hard to define (McCormack and McCance 2010). David considered looking at practical things, such as whether more individualized seating arrangements and activity programmes are now provided. However, while these are important, he wants to evaluate whether the ethos of care provision and the everyday interactions that underpin practice are now more person centred than they were. In trying to articulate what it is he wants to evaluate and how he will know if it is happening, he has come across McCormack and McCance's (2010) four outcomes of person-centred care:

- satisfaction with care
- involvement with care
- feeling of wellbeing
- creating a therapeutic culture.

David thinks these will be a useful way of articulating what he is looking for as the intended outcomes of his CMO process.

David initially thought that the first outcome of interest, satisfaction with care, could be difficult to evaluate, as it requires satisfaction and its features to be defined (McCormack and McCance 2010). However, he has read that satisfaction with care in the context of person-centred practice development can be demonstrated by systems that facilitate shared decision making, effective staff relationships, and professional competence. This latter point refers to moving beyond competence with technical elements of care to include inter-personal skills and working with individual needs (McCormack and McCance 2010). Because practice development methodology stresses the importance of recognizing the personhood of all the people involved, David thinks his eval-uation of these indicators of satisfaction will need to include the perspectives of staff, residents and residents' families.

Practice pointer 9.5

Satisfaction with care may be evaluated by assessing whether:

- systems that are in place facilitate shared decision making
- staff relationships are effective
- professionals are competent (McCormack and McCance 2010).

The second outcome of person-centred care, evidence of involvement with care, includes staff having well-developed interpersonal skills and commit-ment to their work. It also encompasses organizational issues, such as an appropriate skill mix, sharing of power, and systems that are supportive of person-centred care (McCormack and McCance 2010).

Practice pointer 9.6

Involvement with care may be evaluated by assessing whether:

- interpersonal skills are well developed
- people show commitment to their work
- the skill mix is appropriate
- there is evidence that power is shared
- the organizational systems support person-centred care (McCormack and McCance 2010).

The third indicator of person-centredness is a sense of wellbeing (McCor-mack and McCance 2010). This includes the physical and emotional health of residents and staff, but also the things that contribute to them having a sense of wellbeing and safety. For example, individual staff and the team as a whole should be clear about their beliefs and values, be able to develop self-knowledge, and work in an environment where they feel able to innovate and take the risks that allow them to deliver person-centred care (McCormack and McCance 2010). David can see how processes such as reflection and crit-ical companionship can assist in achieving this, and therefore why evidence of staff engaging in these will be indicators that more person-centred care has the chance to develop.

Practice pointer 9.7

A sense of wellbeing may be evaluated by assessing whether:

- people's physical and emotional health needs are met
- practitioners feel able to engage in innovation and risk taking
- practitioners are clear about their beliefs and values
- practitioners are engaged in developing self-knowledge (McCormack and McCance 2010).

Finally, McCormack and McCance (2010) cite the existence of a therapeutic culture as an outcome of interest in person-centred care. This includes practitioners feeling empowered, being autonomous, accountable and reflective, using evidence to inform practice, working with patients' beliefs and values, providing for patients' physical needs, sharing decision making, having sympathetic presence, and being engaged with patients. David can see that these link not only to the thinking processes involved in developing practice, such as supportive challenging, critical reflection and reflexivity, but to visible outcomes in terms of the care provided for residents.

Practice pointer 9.8

The existence of a therapeutic culture may be evaluated by assessing whether:

- practitioners feel empowered
- practitioners act with autonomy
- practitioners are accountable and reflective
- evidence is used to inform practice
- practitioners focus on working with patients' beliefs and values
- practitioners meet patients' physical needs
- there is shared decision making
- patients experience a sympathetic presence from practitioners
- practitioners are engaged with patients (McCormack and McCance 2010).

In addition to these four outcomes, if an intended consequence of developing practice is to create a learning culture, as described in Chapter 4, the degree to which this has been achieved and how it has been approached also needs to be evaluated (Holma and Kontinen 2011). For a learning culture consistent with practice development methodology to be evident, David thinks that people being critically reflective and appraising of themselves and others, and mechanisms being in place to help them achieve this will need to be evident (Manley et al. 2013b).

David believes that using these five categories will enable him to focus the evaluation on outcomes related to the mechanisms that have been put in place to develop more person-centred care. However, he can also see overlaps between each category, the outcomes within it, and how they may be demonstrated. He has therefore grouped the outcomes from across all five categories into particular themes, which he thinks he will use to structure the practicalities of evaluating of person-centred care in his workplace. This will help him to determine how to evaluate them, avoid duplicating information, but also ensure that nothing is missed. Box 9.1 shows how he has grouped the outcomes into themes.

Box 9.1 How David grouped the outcomes and themes he would use to evaluate person-centred practice

Theme: systems
Appropriate skill mix, systems that facilitate shared decision making, organizational systems that are supportive of person-centred care, mechanisms to help teams reflectively discuss situations, structures to support lifelong learning

Outcomes: involvement with care, satisfaction with care, learning culture

Theme: staff relationships
Effective staff relationships, open, honest and clear communication, the contributions that all members make in their roles is recognized

Outcomes: satisfaction with care, learning culture

Theme: physical care
Competence with care, providing for physical needs

Outcomes: satisfaction with care, existence of a therapeutic culture

Theme: interpersonal skills
Competence in communication, evidence of developed interpersonal skills by staff

Outcomes: satisfaction with care, involvement with care

Theme: seeing the individual
Working with individual needs, working with patients' beliefs and values, having sympathetic presence, engagement

Outcomes: satisfaction with care, existence of a therapeutic culture

Theme: commitment to work

Commitment to the job, engagement

Outcome: involvement with care

Theme: power issues

Staff feeling and being able to engage in innovation and risk taking, empowered, autonomous and accountable practitioners, sharing of power, sharing decision making

Outcomes: a sense of wellbeing, involvement with care, existence of a therapeutic culture

Theme: self-knowledge

Clarity over beliefs and values, developing self-knowledge, reflective practitioners, ability to self-appraise

Outcomes: sense of wellbeing, existence of a therapeutic culture, learning culture

Theme: use of evidence

Use of evidence in practice, ability to link theory with practice through reflective conversations

Outcomes: existence of a therapeutic culture, learning culture

Evaluation design and methods

Having decided what he needs to evaluate, David has used the themes shown in Box 9.1 to help him to decide on the methods he will need to use to achieve this. Some of these methods are likely to draw on the principles of quantitative research, because he wants to measure facts (McGrath and Johnson 2003, Lee 2006). However, he will also need to explore people's personal experiences, views, attitudes and values, and thinks that using the principles of qualitative research will be useful in this respect (Kearney 2005, Reid et al. 2007, Rycroft-Malone et al. 2009).

David therefore plans to use a mix of methods to evaluate the developments in practice in his workplace. This fits the principles of realistic evaluation, in which Pommier et al. (2010) and Pedersen et al. (2012) suggest that quantitative methods, qualitative methods, or a combination of these can be used, depending on what is being evaluated. Using a mix of methods is valuable as it allows different aspects of situations to be explored and the reasons for the success or otherwise of various approaches to be investigated (Garbarino and Holland 2009). As well as the principles of realistic evaluation, David therefore thinks he may draw on the principles of mixed methods research (Creswell 2003, Tashakkori and Teddlie 2003, Mertens 2005, Curry et al. 2009).

The dominant focus in realistic evaluation is often on qualitative information, because of the need to explore individual circumstances, views, beliefs, priorities and influences on situations and actions (Pommier et al. 2010). However, David also thinks that quantification of issues such as staffing levels, skill mix, number of agency staff used, and attendance at reflective sessions will give him useful information about how systems support, or do not support, person-centred care. Using qualitative and quantitative information together is also likely to provide a more complete picture of events than each would of itself. For example, if people say they want to attend reflective sessions, but there are never enough staff for them to do so, David can use the rotas to determine staffing trends and what the staffing levels have been on particular occasions.

Practice pointer 9.9

The approach to gathering evaluative evidence should match the nature of what is being evaluated. This may include qualitative approaches, quantitative approaches or a mix of these.

Although qualitative approaches are likely to dominate in David's evaluation, the sequence in which he collects information will also be important. He has decided to use a sequential approach, in which he will gather the quantitative information first, followed by the qualitative data. His rationale is that this will enable him to use the quantified information to inform discussions and consider areas that might require further exploration. However, his initial design needs to be flexible, depending on the information he obtains. For example, the qualitative information may highlight that it would be beneficial for him to gather additional quantifiable evidence.

Having decided on the design of his evaluation, David has to select the tools he will use to evaluate the development of person-centred care. He is considering using a range of approaches, shown in Box 9.2, but the dominant method will be discussions with the key people involved. Discussions seem to David to be a better method than questionnaires, because they will probably enable him to seek more in-depth information about what works, what does not and why this is so. He is planning to use semi-structured discussions, because these will enable the dialogue to be flexible according to what is said and the things individuals feel are important, but still remain focused on the development of person-centred care. Sometimes, an innovation in practice has unexpected outcomes and therefore evaluation strategies need to be flexible enough to identify these (Reed and Turner 2005). One advantage of using semi-structured discussions is that these will allow David to engage in relevant but unplanned areas of discussion.

Box 9.2 Methods used to evaluate the development of person-centred care

Systems
Evaluate using: Quantitative data: numbers on staff rota (including sickness/absence/use of agency staff), numbers attending reflective sessions (frequency and who attended); qualitative data: one-to-one discussions with staff, reflective notes

Staff relationships
Evaluate using: Qualitative data: one-to-one discussions with staff, residents and families, reflective notes

Physical care
Evaluate using: Quantitative data: incident forms; qualitative data: one-to-one discussions with staff, residents and families, reflective notes

Interpersonal skills
Evaluate using: Qualitative data: one-to-one discussions with staff, residents and families, reflective notes

Seeing the individual
Evaluate using: Qualitative data: one-to-one discussions with staff, residents and families, reflective notes

Commitment to work
Evaluate using: Qualitative data: one-to-one discussions with staff, residents and families, reflective notes

Power issues
Evaluate using: Qualitative data: one-to-one discussions with staff, residents and families, reflective notes

Self-knowledge
Evaluate using: Qualitative data: one-to-one discussions with staff, residents and families, reflective notes

Use of evidence
Evaluate using: Qualitative data: one-to-one discussions with staff, residents and families, reflective notes

---

David also wants to be able to capture any differences between rhetoric, intentions, beliefs and what actually happens (Haveri 2008). This is particularly key in evaluating developments in practice, because what happens, rather than what people think should happen, is what matters. In addition, because critical realism acknowledges that actions and interpretations are contextually influenced, David needs to be able to identify whether people are able to do as they intend, or want, to do, and how different people perceive what is done. The methods he is planning to use therefore include discussions in which different perspectives can be seen and intention and achievement noted. For example, if staff feel that they have embraced a more person-centred approach, but residents and families do not experience this, the discussions may be able to shed light on why these different perspectives exist.

Introducing person-centred care is not the only major event in the home at this point in time. David therefore wants to use methods that can distinguish between what is happening because of the new way of working and things that are happening at the same time but are nothing to do with the process of developing person-centred practice. These may include staffing levels and other organizational changes or competing priorities such as the refurbishment (Blamey and Mackenzie 2007). By using in-depth discussions, he hopes to be able to unpick the complexity of everything influencing the development of person-centred care, and explore what are, and what are not, its outcomes.

The type of information David wants to gather could be obtained by holding one-to-one or group discussions. Individual discussions have the advantage that people will not be constrained by what others might think or say, and will be able to enter into a deep discussion about their own perspectives. However, group discussions also have merits: they allow individuals to remind each other of key events, build on each other's responses, and enable group processes, which are an important part of understanding what influences decisions, to be noted. On balance, David has decided that he will aim to hold individual discussions with a sample of residents, relatives of residents and staff.

David has kept a record of his own experiences, observations, thoughts and reflections throughout the process of his team beginning to develop person-centred practice. These include informal conversations and observations that provide him with insights about the implementation of person-centred care, but also things he thinks could influence how he interprets the evaluative information that is gathered. For example, he has noted the occasion on which the owner of the home commented to him: 'I'm looking forward to seeing the improvements you've made in care here.' He recorded this conversation because he wants to guard against being biased in his evaluation because of the owner's expectations. David therefore now intends to use his reflections as a part of the evaluation data (Skinner 2004, Reed and Turner 2005).

Activity 9.3

How could you design an evaluation to capture what people do as well as what they intend to do or say they do, and any unexpected outcomes of developing person-centred care?

Practice pointer 9.10

Evaluation methods should:

- accurately and fully capture the type of information sought
- capture any possible differences between rhetoric and reality
- enable the reasons for outcomes to be explored
- be open to unexpected outcomes.

In some instances, everyone or everything involved can be included in the information gathered for evaluation purposes. David is planning to look at all the rotas and numbers attending reflective sessions over the first six months of the new initiative and this part of his evaluation will therefore use the whole available sample during that time span. However, where the entire population of events or people cannot be used in an evaluation, how the participants or events to be included will be selected is important.

David wants to gain the views of as many people as possible, but thinks it will be unrealistic to try to gain the depth of information he needs from all staff, residents and families. So, he needs to decide how to select people to participate in the evaluative discussions.

One choice open to David is to select people by using probability sampling, in which each resident, relative and staff member has an equal chance of being included in the sample chosen. This usually involves randomization and is often seen as the best approach in quantitative enquiry, where the intention is to provide generalizable results; hence, the need for there to be an equal chance of anyone from the population studied being selected. However, it is not usually used in qualitative enquiry, where the intention is to explore in some depth the particular perspectives of individuals. The aspect of evaluation in which David thinks he will not be able to include everyone is the part that aims to gather qualitative information, so he decides that probability sampling will not be the right approach. Instead, he plans to use a form of non-probability sampling, where not everyone has an equal chance of being selected and randomization is not used.

David may use purposive sampling, a form of non-probability sampling where participants are chosen deliberately, sometimes because they have a particular experience or are likely to have a particular way of viewing a situation (Astin 2009). Although this can be a useful approach, it means that some people will not be invited to share their views because they are not chosen. Another option is for David to use a volunteer sample, where an invitation is issued to the entire population and those who want to participate volunteer. A benefit of this approach is that those who volunteer are likely to be interested in what is being evaluated and willing to participate. A downside is that those who have positive things to report and those who have negative perspectives are likely to volunteer, but people whose opinions are relatively neutral are less likely to be represented. It also means that those who lack the confidence to volunteer will be missed. These and other approaches to selecting a sample for evaluation have benefits and problems, which have to be weighed up.

David thinks he will probably use a mix of volunteer and purposive sampling. He will begin by asking for volunteers who are prepared to share their thoughts and experiences. However, if someone who volunteers to participate makes him aware of a person with a particular experience whose views it would be useful to have, he will ask them if they would like to participate in the evaluation, even though they have not volunteered. He may, therefore, also use a form of what is known as snowball sampling, where one participant refers the person conducting the evaluation to other potential participants.

It is often necessary to decide between the ideal and the manageable. When evaluation information is analysed, the decisions that were made about sampling will influence the way findings are interpreted and the confidence with which any recommendations are made. If, for example, David decides that he will, for practical reasons, only hold discussions with relatives who visit frequently, he will need to note that the evaluation did not include how relatives who visit infrequently and those who predominantly stay in touch by telephone perceive care.

Practice pointer 9.11

- Evaluating person-centred practice usually involves gathering information from people.
- Decisions have to be made about which groups of people information will be gathered from and which people within those groups will be asked to participate.

Activity 9.4

What sample of people or events would you use to evaluate person-centred care in your workplace?

Who should evaluate

The person or people who conduct an evaluation can affect its quality (Skinner 2004). This includes whether the person collecting the information will affect what people say or do, and if they will influence how the information is interpreted and analysed (Comfort 2010). As Chapter 5 identified, practice development methodology sees incorporating those who are the recipients of care in the process of developing practice as vital and David wants to involve staff, relatives and residents in collecting evaluative information. However, it is also important that people are prepared for their role and want to be involved, rather than feeling coerced to participate. While David wants residents and their relatives to be a part of evaluating the development of person-centred practice, he needs to ensure that they are involved in activities in which they felt confident and comfortable. He wonders, for example, if the residents who have been involved in the process of developing person-centred care will feel comfortable holding one-to-one evaluative discussions, and thinks instead that their key role may be in helping to analyse the information that has been gathered. He intends to discuss the different roles in the evaluation process and what they will involve with the group he has worked with on developing person-centred practice, so that each individual can choose what they would prefer to do.

As well as people's skills and confidence, the evaluation has to be conducted by people who have enough time and commitment to do the necessary work (Comfort 2010). David therefore plans to outline to the group what each stage of the evaluation will involve, when he expects it to happen, and what it will require in terms of people's time.

David is also considering how the identity of those conducting the evaluation may influence the findings. He knows that it may be hard for him to be unbiased about the new way of working, because it was his idea, and he has put time and effort into it. He also feels some pressure from the owner of the home to demonstrate that the team are now working in a person-centred way, which may make it difficult for him to be completely unbiased. He hopes that using a variety of people to collect and analyse the information and the emergent findings being discussed by the group as a whole will reduce the effect of his potential biases.

Activity 9.5

Who would you use to conduct an evaluation of person-centred care in your workplace?

When to evaluate

Practice development methodology includes processes of almost continuous reflection and evaluation. However, it is also useful to have formal points at which progress is checked. David thinks that six months into the process is a reasonable time to formally take stock and consider the team's journey so far, what could be built on and developed further, and what might need rethinking. However, as Chapter 10 will discuss, he also thinks that, as time goes by, people's enthusiasm for developing person-centred care may lessen, other priorities come along, and people revert to previous practices and habits (Balasubramanian et al. 2010). To pick up on whether this is happening and enable developments in practice to continue to be celebrated and further refined, David is planning ongoing evaluations. The second will be one year after the beginning of the initiative, followed by evaluations at yearly intervals.

Practice pointer 9.12

The timing of evaluations should be planned so as to allow enough time to show the effects of a new way of working, frequent enough that things are not missed but not so frequent as to distract from the development itself, and over a long enough period to sustain developments.

Analysing the evidence from evaluation activities

A part of planning an evaluation is deciding how the information gleaned will be analysed. The numerical information that David collects will need to be dealt with using numerical means. As the numbers used will be small, David anticipates using descriptive statistics in the form of raw scores and percentages (Windish and Diener-West 2006). This is usually completely acceptable in evaluating developments in practice, because the sample is unlikely to be large enough to do otherwise, and the intention is to see how things have worked out in the environment in question, not to generalize the findings. Inferential statistics are only appropriate if the scale or intention of the evaluation merits it. Measurements in any evaluation should be valid and accurate, suitable for the issue in question, but not unnecessarily complex (Harvey and Wensing 2003).

For the qualitative information, David plans to have the recordings and notes taken during discussions transcribed and to code these, and his reflective notes, into key ideas, then arrange these codes into larger categories or themes (Burla et al. 2008, Balls 2009, Campos and Turato 2009).

Respondent validation is often used in qualitative enquiry to check that the interpretations of the person carrying out data analysis are consistent with what participants intended to convey (Koch 2006, Roberts and Priest 2006). Nonetheless, although this is generally considered to be a good way of checking the accuracy of qualitative information, it can present difficulties if the interpretations of the person analysing the conversations and that of participants is significantly different. It is therefore useful to decide in advance what level of interpretation participants will be invited to comment on, for example whether they will be asked to check that the transcript of a discussion accurately reflects what they said and felt, or whether they will be invited to comment on the interpretation of this information. David plans to check with those involved in discussions that what they said has been accurately interpreted. He thinks that practice development's emphasis on mutual respect between people and recognition of different perceptions of reality lends itself to discussing any differences in the interpretation of information, with such dialogue becoming a part of the evaluative data.

Because the evaluation David is planning will include various types of information, these will need to be brought together into a meaningful whole. David will also need to link the findings to the five areas of person-centredness he has identified (see Box 9.1), and place these into the CMO model he has developed. David is not exactly sure how fitting the information he gathers into the five categories and CMO model will work, because this is largely dependent on the findings. There may be clear links, or links that are not so clear, between the C, M and O and between particular aspects of the CMO and the five outcomes of practice development. For instance, David recently heard a member of staff discussing with a resident why she was unable to help her to get her hair done. His reflections on this discussion could, he realized, relate to the context, but also the mechanisms that have been put in place to try to develop person-centred care. Equally, it might concern the systems put in place to enable person-centred care, or the individual's commitment to their work. Jackson and Kolla (2012) found that putting the findings from realistic evaluation together can be a complex process, with people's discussions often almost inextricably linking context, mechanism and outcome in single units of dialogue. Knowing this has guided David to develop a timescale for evaluation that includes enough time for in-depth exploration of the information gathered, its meaning and how it fits together. He is also mindful that he is using the principles of realistic evaluation, not necessarily realistic evaluation in its entirety, and should work with the information produced, and remain true to this, rather than trying to force it to fit a particular model or approach.

> **Practice pointer 9.13**
>
> • Analysis of the information gathered in evaluation activities should match the type of information gathered.
> • If more than one type of information is being gathered, how the different types of information will be put together to make a whole picture has to be decided.

Ethics and evaluation

The ethical obligation healthcare staff have to do good and to do no harm means that introducing new practice without evaluating its outcome could be considered unethical, as the effect of the innovation and whether it is a valid use of resources are unknown (Hughes 2008). Although developing more person-centred care seems likely to be beneficial, David considers it important to check that this is indeed so.

When new practice is evaluated, there is also an ethical obligation to obtain and present as accurate as possible a picture of events, so that the recommendations made for ongoing practice are a true reflection of the benefits and challenges of the innovation.

> **Practice pointer 9.14**
>
> Evaluation of any practice development initiative should follow the principles of healthcare ethics.

Evaluation activities should comply with ethical principles. However, an evaluation of an innovation in practice will not usually require approval by an ethics committee, as it involves something of which evaluation is the natural conclusion, rather than an activity for its own end (NPSA/NRES 2009). It is more common for the process of developing practice, including evaluative activities, to be approved through local governance processes. The way in which the evaluation of developments in practice is conducted should nonetheless follow the principles of healthcare ethics in terms of respecting autonomy, doing good, doing no harm, and seeking justice (Beauchamp and Childress 2008). In terms of benefit and harm, the fate of developing person-centred care in his workplace largely rests on the findings from David's evaluation. Therefore, the findings from the evaluation need to be a true and accurate representation of the effects of the new system, so that if it is beneficial, it will be developed further, and if not, it can be modified or discontinued. However, it is also important to consider the benefits and harms for individuals who are involved in the evaluation. People may derive a benefit from participating in this process, and having their views heard. However, harm may occur if they feel coerced to participate, uncomfortable about expressing their views, or that their work is being unnecessarily scrutinized. They may also be disappointed if they believe the evaluation will bring outcomes that do not then materialize.

The principle of respect for autonomy in relation to evaluation concerns the degree of choice that individuals or groups have about participating in an evaluation, and whether they give informed consent for this (Coughlan et al. 2007). David is in a relatively senior position, and staff, residents and relatives could feel coerced to participate in the evaluation, obliged to give positive responses about the development of person-centred care, or constrained to allow their discussions to be audio recorded when they would prefer them not to be. David therefore needs to take steps to minimize the risk of this being the case, and to ensure that the consent people give to participate is fully informed and freely given.

Meeting the ethical requirement for justice includes whether everyone has an equal chance to contribute to or be represented in the evaluation activities. David feels that this will be achieved by using a volunteer sample. However, if everyone volunteers, he may need to develop a fair and transparent way of deciding who will have the chance to participate.

Activity 9.6

What ethical issues would you need to consider in evaluating person-centred care in your workplace?

Summary

David considers evaluating the development of person-centred practice in his workplace important. Although he and his team are engaged in continuous, reflective processes, he thinks it will be beneficial to have formal points at which stock is taken and decisions made as to what is and is not working and why this is, so that what is good can be maintained and what is less good reviewed and adjusted. This has links to the cycles of action research seen in practice development methodology.

Evaluation of practice development should be designed to fit the ethos that underpins the whole activity. David thinks that the principles of realistic evaluation may be useful in this respect, as it has links with person-centredness, critical social theory and critical realism. However, its original form may need to be adapted to accommodate the complex and somewhat imprecise nature of developing person-centred care.

Within these principles, David aims to use methods of collecting and analysing information that are focused on the development and delivery of a person-centred work ethos, and are systematic, rigorous and consistent with the ethical principles of healthcare. In the longer term, David plans to use the findings from this and ongoing evaluations as a part of sustaining a culture of person-centred working.

Case scenario

Yvonne is the ward manager of an acute mental health ward. She came into post 18 months ago and has been working with her team to develop a more person-centred approach to care. The idea was not met with enthusiasm and the development process has been slow. However, she believes that progress has been made, and is now considering how to evaluate the developments that have taken place to date.

Whose experiences and perspectives will Yvonne need to explore?

Yvonne thinks she needs to explore the experiences and perspectives of people who have been admitted to the ward and the staff who have cared for them. The staff aspect will mainly focus on nurses, as they are the group who have been most involved in this initiative. Yvonne believes that investigating the perspectives of medical staff, psychologists, occupational therapists and other members of the multidisciplinary team who visit the ward regularly would also be interesting. However, she is planning to leave this until the next evaluation, by which time she hopes that person-centred care will be more firmly established and showing more outcomes that other professions would notice. She also expects that non-nursing staff will have become a part of the reflective groups by that stage. One of the occupational therapists has recently joined in and she thinks others may follow. Nonetheless, she wants the evaluation to be manageable and focus on what has happened to date, not what she hopes to achieve in the future.

Although Yvonne wants to seek patients' perspectives, she can see problems with doing this while they are still on the ward. She therefore plans to seek their views at the point of discharge home, or soon afterwards.

Yvonne ultimately wants to explore the experiences of patients' families, particularly their partners or those who provide their main support in the community. However, she has decided to leave this until a later evaluation, when person-centred care is more developed.

The context of Yvonne's workplace

Yvonne works on a 20-bed ward, where people aged 16 and above are admitted because of acute mental health conditions. Most of the staff have worked there for many years, and although new members of staff have been appointed from time to time, they have seldom stayed for longer than a few months. When Yvonne arrived in post, the mainstay of activities for patients was receiving specific interventions, watching TV, reading magazines and newspapers, or being seen by specialist staff. The ward was focused on routines, with the activities of staff and patients based on tasks that needed to be accomplished. Staff often sat in the lounge with patients, but interactions between them were not very purposeful, despite being mainly perfectly amicable.

Initially, the idea of looking towards providing a more person-centred approach to care was not popular. However, the nursing staff have gradually begun to engage with the process, and it seems to Yvonne that many of them now view the opportunity to work in a different way positively. There are two particularly strong characters on the ward, both of whom opposed the idea of more person-centred working and are people who other staff members tend to listen to. However, over time, their influence appears to be lessening, even though their opposition is not. Although there are no obvious changes in how the ward is organized, Yvonne has noticed more meaningful interactions when staff sit in the lounge with patients, and when they are working one to one with them. She frequently hears conversations that indicate a genuine interest in people, in a way that she did not before. In reflective sessions, practitioners are becoming more inclined to think about what they do, how they interact with patients, and to challenge themselves and one another.

How could Yvonne design an evaluation to capture what people do as well as what they intend to do or say they do, and any unexpected outcomes of developing person-centred care?

Yvonne is designing an evaluation that predominantly uses qualitative approaches to gathering information to gain an in-depth understanding of how people perceive their work, how they intend to work, whether they find they can do this in practice, and their views on this. She aims to achieve this by conducting group discussions with nursing staff. Using group rather than one-to-one discussions has the downside that some group members may dominate, and people may feel obliged to conform to what others say. However, as the team are becoming familiar with reflective group discussions, she thinks that this downside will be minimal. Using a group approach will also enable her to see if there is any evidence of peer pressure for people to conform to certain views, which might influence the enactment of person-centred care. It will also mean, practically, that she can include all those who wish to participate in the evaluation.

Yvonne plans to hold one-to-one discussions with patients to explore their perspectives on the care they have received. In addition, she has noted her own reflections and perceptions during the process of developing person-centred care, and intends to compare these, staff and patients' perspectives.

Yvonne has introduced a comments box on the ward, in which staff, patients and visitors can post their views and suggestions. She thinks the comments made could be a useful addition to the evaluation data.

Yvonne also thinks that some quantification of events will be helpful. For example, to identify how many reflective sessions have been held, how many people have attended them, and how this links to staffing levels, bed occupancy and patient dependency levels. She believes that while her greatest focus will be on the qualitative information, quantitative evidence will also be useful to explore and explain some of the 'whys' of what happens, or is perceived to happen. Yvonne is therefore planning to use a mix of methods, but with a strong focus on qualitative information.

How will Yvonne decide on what sample of people or events to use to evaluate person-centred care in her workplace?

Yvonne plans to look at staff rotas, bed occupancy, dependency levels and attendance at reflective sessions over the past year to give a full view of seasonal variations and their effects on events on the ward.

Yvonne wants to capture the views of all the nursing staff, but holding one-to-one discussions with everyone would be too time-consuming. She therefore plans to hold group discussions, which will mean that everyone's views can be captured.

To ascertain patients' views, Yvonne plans to ask all the patients who are discharged over a one-month period if they are prepared to engage in one-to-one discussions about their experiences.

The information provided via the suggestions and feedback box will be a part of the evaluation and will be open for everyone to participate in.

Who will Yvonne use to conduct the evaluation of person-centred care?

Yvonne thinks she will need to lead the evaluation, as she has led the process of developing practice, understands what needs to be evaluated and why. However, she plans to ask someone else to work with her on analysing the rotas, bed occupancy figures, dependency levels, numbers attending reflective sessions, and collating the information from the comments box. As well as sharing the workload and involving people, this may lend more credibility to the evaluation, as she may be considered to have a vested interest in showing that things are working well.

Yvonne has identified one other nurse who is keen on developing more person-centred care and with whom she ultimately hopes to share leadership of the person-centred care initiative. She thinks she could ask this person to help facilitate the discussions with patients.

Yvonne thinks she should facilitate the staff discussions. This may create a risk of bias in that she may lead people to the answers she wants, but equally she is used to working with them in reflective sessions and encouraging people to express their views. She knows the sort of thing she wants to find out about, not just in terms of people's use of person-centred care, but also the factors that enable or detract from it. She may therefore be the person best placed to keep discussions focused on the key issues for the evaluation. However, she intends to ask the person she sees as a potential future leader to co-facilitate these groups, to balance her own views and input, and to prepare her colleague for taking on a greater role in the development of person-centred practice.

What ethical issues will Yvonne need to consider in evaluating person-centred care?

Yvonne is aware that the patients whose views she will be seeking are a potentially vulnerable group. They may feel coerced, or obliged, to give positive reports on their experiences, and be fearful that any perceived criticism might be detrimental to their future care. She has considered asking an outside person to hold the discussions with them, but this also has challenges, in terms of practicalities, funding and their knowledge of the aims of the developments in practice. She thinks she will conduct the discussions, but will be clear in her explanations, verbally and in writing, that no one is obliged to participate, people's identities will be kept confidential in any feedback, and as the intention is to improve services, she wants to hear what is not good as well as positives.

Staff may similarly feel coerced to participate, obliged to give the responses they feel Yvonne wants to hear, or concerned about disclosing anything that might be considered poor practice. Again, Yvonne will seek to assure them that the ground rules of confidentiality they are used to in reflective work will apply. Her emphasis will be that she wants to know what works but also what does not, and that it is important to know both in order to effectively improve things for patients, but also staff. Although she ideally wants to speak to all staff, no one will be obliged to participate.

In terms of justice, all staff will be invited to participate. While not all patients will be invited to discuss their experiences, everyone in a particular time frame will be, and written comments from everyone who has made them will be used. The limitation of a given time frame is a necessary practicality, but also because Yvonne wants to capture the most recent experiences so that the evaluation is up to date.

Yvonne has sought approval for the evaluation through the local clinical governance group.

Additional resources

Evaluation tools and methods
http://evaluationtoolbox.net.au/index.php?option=com_content&view=article&id=51&Itemid=131
Provides suggestions on which tools to use in different circumstances.

Realistic evaluation
http://etheses.bham.ac.uk/237/1/Thistleton08EdD.pdf
A doctoral thesis that used realistic evaluation.

www.worcestershire.gov.uk/cms/pdf/Realistic%20Evaluation%20(2).pdf
An example of how realistic evaluation can be used.

Evaluating person-centred care
www.pifonline.org.uk/tools-for-evaluating-and-measuring-person-centred-care
Provides tools for evaluating person-centred care.

www.health.org.uk/public/cms/75/76/313/4697/Helping%20measure%20person-centred%20care.pdf?realName=Inet6X.pdf
Health Foundation's review of commonly used approaches to and tools for measuring person-centred care.

www.science.ulster.ac.uk/inhr/pcp/resources.php
Provides information about and links to McCormack and McCance's Person-centred Nursing Index and Slater and McCormack's Person-centred Caring Index.

Evaluating practice development
www.canterbury.ac.uk/health/documents/ouctomesandmultipleagendas.pdf
Position paper on the need for a strategic level evaluation framework for practice development.

10 Maintaining a Culture of Person-centred Practice Development

Chapter overview

- Putting in place mechanisms to sustain developments in practice is as important as making the initial developments.
- The greatest threat to sustaining a culture of person-centred care is that it is slowly eroded by other priorities and demands.
- Measures that can assist in sustaining person-centred practice include:
  - linking new innovations and requirements to this ethos
  - highlighting ongoing developments and their benefits
  - being alert to losses that may accrue and develop over time
  - being aware of anyone who continues to oppose this way of working
  - succession planning
  - securing continued resources and managerial buy-in
  - preparing new staff for this approach
  - continuing to provide, seek and act on feedback.

Husna works on a children's medical ward. About 18 months ago, she began to think that although her ward practised what was described as family-centred care, it was not really person centred, in terms of placing the people concerned and their particular and individual needs centrally (McCormack et al. 2009). She and her colleagues were generally friendly, approachable and tried to meet families' needs. However, they did not seem to Husna to consistently work in a way that acknowledged each person's uniqueness and sought to view things from their perspective (Parish 2012). 'Partnership in care' was often referred to, but Husna did not think this achieved the equality of status and mutual collaboration that constitutes person-centredness (McCormack et al. 2010, McKay et al. 2012, van den Pol-Grevelink et al. 2012). As a result, over the past year or so, she has been using the principles of practice development methodology to try to develop a more child and family-centred culture on the ward. This has primarily involved the use of reflective discussions and critical companionship, as described in Chapter 4. These processes have been led by an external facilitator, who has also sought to develop the skills of facilitation in the ward staff, so that they become self-sufficient in this respect (Larsen et al. 2005, Manley et al. 2013b). The facilitator still runs some reflective groups, but the staff themselves now largely manage their own reflective activities and critical companionship. Initially, only the nursing staff were involved in this process, but in the last three months, two of the medical staff and a physiotherapist have joined the reflective groups.

In line with the importance of involving the recipients of care in developing person-centred practice, families have been instrumental in the process of developing child and family-centred care on Husna's ward (McCormack et al. 2006). Deciding how to involve families presented some challenges (as outlined in Chapter 5), but two parents whose children have been cared for on the ward often attend reflective sessions to share insights and reflect on their own experiences and perceptions. One of these parents is the father of a child with a long-term condition who has ongoing admissions to the ward.

Husna thinks the care the ward provides is now much more centred on children and their families as individual people with specific priorities and needs outside their medical requirements. She also believes that both staff and parents seem more satisfied with care provision. As part of the process of developing practice, there have been four specific changes in the way things are done on the ward:

- how parents' nutrition needs are catered for
- how regulations on parents staying overnight are interpreted
- the regulations about the numbers of visitors permitted
- how nursing staff are allocated to care for families.

However, the key change is that the ethos of care is more focused on knowing the children and families as individuals, and tailoring interactions, provision and care to this.

While things seem to have gone well, Husna is aware that not everyone was convinced at the outset that making a specific effort to enable care to become more child and family centred was necessary. Two members of staff stated from the beginning that the ward already practised family-centred care, and therefore developing a more person-centred approach was unnecessary. They argued that the time taken for this would detract from the direct care that children needed, and could interfere with the smooth running of the ward. Another of Husna's colleagues considered the developments to be rather 'fluffy', with no real evidence of what benefit there would be for the effort put in. A fourth person has never really shown interest in, or engaged with, the process. Husna thinks that while these people do not appear to have detracted from the progress made to date, they could still be influential. She is also aware that while everyone else seems to think the culture has now changed for the better, it would not take much for things to slowly slide back to how they were before.

Husna's reservations are justified. Many changes in practice are initially successful but are not sustained over time (Virani et al. 2009). The development that Husna has led is different from changing a particular aspect of practice, but it may still become something that was good while it lasted, but not sustained long term. As Chapter 1 identified, a workplace culture is not a static entity, but is constantly evolving (Jordan 2009). Thus, while the culture on Husna's ward has become more child and family centred, it would be easy for it to move back to being tokenistically so. While devoting time, energy and resources to developing a more child and family-centred approach to care has been vital, Husna is convinced that it is now equally crucial for efforts to be made to sustain this over time.

Practice pointer 10.1

Successful developments in practice may not be sustained over time unless an ongoing effort is made to continue to develop them.

Although the time when a new initiative is being developed and introduced is often where the focus is, efforts are also required to sustain it over time and enable it to become embedded in practice (Virani et al. 2009). Husna considers this to be true of the development of a more child and family-centred culture. She initially devoted a lot of time and effort to discussing the idea with people, working with those who were less certain, and setting up the necessary processes for it to happen. Over time, people have come on board, disciplines other than nursing are now involved, and the majority of Husna's colleagues seem to enjoy working in this way and are proud of it. However, if this culture of child and family-centred care is to be sustained, the initial efforts that have been made need to continue.

Practice pointer 10.2

Culture is not a static entity: developing a more person-centred culture can be followed by a return to a less person-centred culture unless efforts are made to sustain the new ethos.

Avoiding a slow slide

Husna considers it unlikely that using a child and family-centred approach to care will be officially stopped, or that those who have adopted this way of working will consciously decide to abandon it. Like all change initiatives, the greatest threat to sustaining child and family-centred care is that it will slowly be afforded less time, attention and effort and gradually be eroded, until it disappears. The greatest risks to the new culture being maintained are people becoming less vigilant about engaging in reflective, reflexive thinking and about seeking and giving supportive but challenging feedback. Husna wants to keep these processes as a central part of the ward's activities so as to maintain the momentum of child and family-centred working (Hall and Hord 2011).

The key elements of developing a more child and family-centred culture on Husna's ward have been:

- using reflective activities (Peek et al. 2007, Dewing 2010, Brown and McCormack 2011)
- high challenge/high support facilitation (McCormack et al. 2009, Manley et al. 2009, Titchen et al. 2013)
- involving families as well as staff in the process of developing person-centred care (McCormack et al. 2006).

Husna thinks it unlikely that many people will intentionally neglect these developments in how they work. They may feel, however, even subconsciously, that as they have now achieved the goal of establishing a more child and family-centred culture, attending reflective groups is not such a priority. Equally, they may, especially when they are busy, fail to give feedback to one another, because they assume that, now things are well established, they can occasionally let it go. This will be an easy trap to fall into, but the risk is that one-off occasions will become more and more frequent and that what has been achieved will slowly drift away. Husna thinks she needs to maintain a focus on the importance of these activities, by role modelling them in her own work and encouraging others to continue to value them, even during busy times.

Practice pointer 10.3

The most common reason for changes in practice not being sustained is that as things become less novel, less time and effort are devoted to them, people become less vigilant and enthusiastic, and practice slowly slides back to how it was before.

Competing priorities

To be sustainable, a development in practice has to be able to withstand the challenges and competing demands that occur over time. These include the competing priorities of everyday care demands and those associated with other, newer innovations or requirements (Buchanan et al. 2005). When Husna first introduced the idea of trying to work in a more child and family-centred way, it was the central activity on the ward. Everyone's attention was on it, and even those who were unsure of its value or opposed it often took the time to comment on it. However, over time, other priorities have developed and there is a risk that attention could move away from the child and family-centred care initiative and things could begin to return to how they were before (Virani et al. 2009, Balasubramanian et al. 2010). The ward is busy, and new policies, procedures or requirements for action are produced regularly. These could move the developments in child and family-centred care further and further down the hierarchy for attention until they are gradually lost. Husna therefore tries to ensure that other changes or developments that come along are incorporated into the culture of child and family-centred care, so that they become a part of, not a competitor with, it.

When new initiatives are suggested or required changes brought to the ward's attention, Husna makes a point of suggesting how they can become a part of child and family-centred care. This means that the new activities are required to fit within this ethos, rather than becoming a challenge to it. For instance, when electronic documentation was introduced, Husna explored how the ward could use this to enhance child and family-centred care provision. Doing so kept the focus on child and family-centred practice, and enabled her remind everyone that this was their core philosophy, within which other developments should be integrated. When other required activities threaten events such as reflective groups, Husna emphasizes their importance so that they are not seen as the thing that can go. Recently, new infusion pumps were being introduced on the ward and the instruction sessions for these were scheduled for a day when a reflective session had been booked. While learning about the new pumps was clearly vital, Husna made a point of ensuring that the ward manager knew they needed to reschedule the reflective event, within a couple of days, and ensured that this happened. This gave a clear message that while she was flexible and understood the competing demands the ward faced, the focus on child and family-centred care would not be the thing that was sacrificed when time was tight.

Activity 10.1

Identify a development in practice you know about that was not sustained. Consider whether competing priorities or newer innovations and demands contributed to this.

Practice pointer 10.4

Competing demands that can erode successful developments in practice include:

- the competing priorities of everyday care
- newer innovations
- new requirements.

A bottom-up approach to change, with developments arising from the insights of frontline practitioners and families, not ideas or requirements from managers, has underpinned the developments on Husna's ward (Manley and McCormack 2003). By continuing to encourage staff and families to identify and work on opportunities to further develop child and family-centred care, Husna intends to keep this process alive and worthy of as much attention and effort as other, newer developments. This also means that it will continue to be owned by staff and families, not Husna, and is something they are a key part of, have invested in and want to maintain because it is theirs.

Although the process of developing practice has been in place for just over a year, Husna is aware that individuals and the team as a whole are still gaining new insights into how day-to-day interactions and care encounters can become more child and family centred. She makes a point of highlighting these to remind her colleagues that this is an ongoing, evolutionary process, with new perceptions that influence everyday care, as well as particular initiatives, still happening regularly. Her intention is to clarify that child and family-centred care is not a goal that has been reached and will now work on its own, but an ongoing journey that is still worth being on.

Practice pointer 10.5

Ways of sustaining a culture of person-centred care include:

- linking newer innovations into the ethos of person-centredness
- exploring how new requirements can be incorporated into the ethos of person-centredness
- highlighting ongoing instances of developments in person-centred care and their benefits
- continuing to emphasize the importance and outcomes of reflective learning.

As well as the risk of people feeling that working in a child and family-centred way will now sustain itself, Husna is aware that those who never really supported this way of working can still sabotage it, especially if no particular effort is made to sustain and develop it.

The risk of detractors influencing others over time

Until a new way of working is fully embedded as a core part of practice, those who have never accepted it can still convince others to revert to how things were before. Husna is fairly sure that some of her colleagues have not really adopted a more child and family-centred way of working. Instead of them eventually deciding to participate, as laggards often do (Rogers 1995, Hall and Hord 2011), they may, over time, convince others to abandon this way of working. They may achieve this by encouraging colleagues to think that missing the odd reflective opportunity or occasionally not spending time getting to know a child and family is not overwhelmingly important, especially when things are busy. If they succeed, over time, more and more opportunities for people to develop their thinking and engage with families will be missed and the ward will slowly regress to the way things were previously.

As Chapter 7 outlined, those who might be described as the late and early majority are the groups whose participation is strongly influenced by the prevailing actions of others (Rogers 1995, Hall and Hord 2011). They are therefore the most likely to be persuaded by the weight of other people's opinions to neglect or abandon a new initiative. Husna knows that if more and more people are seen to be lowering the priority afforded to family-centred care, the late and early majority are likely to follow their lead. If, on the other hand, a strong majority continue to value this, they will probably also continue to work in this way.

One of Husna's strategies to stop those who are not engaged with the new way of working from adversely influencing their colleagues' participation is to avoid any suggestion that the new culture is now achieved and can be left to manage itself (Kotter 1995). Instead, she focuses on giving encouragement, praise and a sense of progress and achievement to her colleagues, while also emphasizing that this is still a work in progress. Giving the impression that everything has now been achieved might enable those who oppose the new way of working to encourage others to think that they no longer need to make an effort. Husna has heard one nurse who she knows has not engaged with developing child and family-centred care say to another nurse: 'You don't need to go to that session, we're busy and that's been done now. You don't need to keep meeting up and talking about it.' If this type of suggestion succeeds, over time, more and more reflective discussions will be missed or person-centred encounters detracted from, and the re-established norm will be how things were before the developments in practice began (Kotter 1995). Despite the importance of celebrating the success of the developments in practice and giving positive feedback on everyone's hard work, Husna also celebrates milestones and the achievement of significant goals, while clarifying that input and effort are still required. She marked the six-month and one-year points from the beginning of the practice development journey by inviting staff to share their experiences, sum up what had changed for them, what they had learned, and presenting evidence from formal evaluations. She also worked with other people on making visual displays about the developments, which were put up on the ward notice boards where staff and families could see them. This enabled the team to celebrate their achievements, but also reminded everyone that this was a work in progress and an expected approach to care. In the reflective sessions and by challenging others in everyday practice and encouraging them to challenge her, Husna also highlights where things have slipped slightly, so that people can see the impact of even a one-off return to a less child and family-centred way of working. This gives the message that while the outcomes of the initiative so far are valuable, she is keeping an eye on things, her efforts are not relaxing and those of her colleagues should not either. She also wants to give a clear message to those who might be wavering that the majority of people are still committed to this way of working.

Practice pointer 10.6

Those who have not embraced person-centred care can still erode this ethos after it is apparently established, by:

- drip-feeding the message that it is not a good idea
- encouraging others to think they can now relax their efforts
- convincing others, one by one, to abandon this way of working.

Activity 10.2

Identify a development in practice you know about that was not sustained (this may be the example used in Activity 10.1). Were there any people who never really supported the innovation in question? Did their influence increase or decrease over time?

At the same time as celebrating the achievements and progress made, Husna is aware that the development of more child and family-centred care may have brought with it losses that could influence whether or not the new way of working is sustained (Price 2008, Hall and Hord 2011).

Ongoing losses

The need to acknowledge and support the losses that any change in prac-tice can bring was highlighted in Chapter 7 (Austin and Currie 2003, Scott et al. 2003, Price 2008, Hall and Hord 2011). As a new way of working contin-ues and becomes established, addressing feelings of loss remains important (Golden 2006). Losses may become less acceptable, rather than diminishing, as time goes by, and people may also encounter losses they had not antici-pated. Those who had hoped that an innovation would not work may realize that it is succeeding, and that the losses they thought they would avoid are becoming real. This may mean that rather than beginning to accept the way things are and participating, they become more resistant and what was passive opposition becomes overt.

Husna realizes that the people who were dismissive of the idea of develop-ing more child and family-centred care generally adopted the stance that this was just another idea that, if ignored, would go away soon enough. However, as it has become clear that this is not the case, their opposition has become a little more obvious and marked. This is possibly due to their disinclination to the idea, and because they now feel loss not just of their comfort in another way of working, but loss of credibility because their cynicism has not been justified. Husna is aware that she needs to focus on not letting their oppo-sition deter others, but also work with them in such a way that they can, if they decide to, still participate in the development of child and family-centred care without it being an embarrassing climb-down. She therefore tries to avoid confrontation with them, and, while keeping a vigilant eye on how their disengagement is affecting others, rarely challenges their actual partici-pation. As well as being a tactic she hopes will work, she feels that a key part of person-centredness is accepting different perspectives, values and viewpoints, and she has to role model this in her dealings with her detractors. She wants to develop a situation wherein they either eventually participate, or decide that the new ethos is not for them and leave the team, rather than her rejecting their perspectives.

As well as existing losses increasing over time, aspects of developments in practice that people had not really considered may begin to cause them to feel loss. Two of the nurses on Husna's ward were always seen as good at working with families. They were among the early adopters and helped to lead the process of developing practice (Rogers 1995, Hall and Hord 2011). Husna has no reason to believe that these two people are other than pleased about the developments in child and family-centred care. Nonetheless, she is aware that their informal role as the experts and the most highly skilled at practising in a child and family-centred way could be eroded as everyone else begins to develop their skills in this way of working. So, she makes a concerted effort to keep them central to the processes in place and encourages them to take evolving leadership roles in developing and maintaining child and family-centred practice.

Practice pointer 10.7

Practice development initiatives may be subject to new challenges over time as the losses people initially felt become more marked, or as new losses they had not considered become apparent.

Activity 10.3

Identify a development in practice you know about that was not sustained (this may be the example used in Activity 10.1). Were there likely to have been any losses associated with this development that developed, increased, or became apparent over time?

Succession planning

As well as the initial leadership of practice development initiatives being important (as discussed in Chapter 8), strong leadership continues to be needed throughout the process. When a development in practice depends on one key leader, if they leave the workplace or are away for a period of time, the initiative and the cultural change associated with it may fail, even after it seems to be established. Husna believes that robust leadership will continue to be needed to sustain the impetus for more child and family-centred care. Although she has led the initial change in practice, she wants to ensure that others are invested in now so as to enable and encourage them to take a lead in the process. Initially, this will probably be alongside her, but, over time, she is looking for other people to take the lead role, and perhaps share this so that it is not dependent on one person. She is therefore nurturing leadership in the two people who were the established experts in working with families, by using some of the ideas discussed in Chapter 8, and arranging for the facilitator to work with them to enable them to develop their leadership skills.

As well as nurturing leadership in key individuals, Husna wants to develop an ethos in which although some people lead the whole process of continuing to develop person-centred care, every person is a leader in a particular way. By creating a culture in which reflection and supportive challenging are the norm, she tries to emphasize that everyone, including the parents who participate, is able and expected to lead others in the process of developing their practice.

Husna is also considering whether, in the longer term, she wants to develop her own role to focus on coaching and developing leadership in others in a way that is congruent with practice development methodology. This will keep her attentive to the overall direction of travel on the ward, while also taking on new challenges and developing new skills herself.

Practice pointer 10.8

• Developing new leaders makes the process of developing and refining person-centred care more sustainable.
• Creating a culture in which everyone is a part of leading the process of person-centred care means that the culture is more likely to be sustained, as it does not depend on one or two key people.

Activity 10.4

Identify a development in practice you know about that was not sustained (this may be the example used in Activity 10.1). Did the way in which leaders were developed influence it not being sustained?

As well as succession planning for the leadership of practice development, Husna has considered how families will remain a central part of developments. One of the parents who is part of the initiative is the father of a child with a long-term condition who is likely to continue to have admissions to the ward. However, the other parent's child is unlikely to be readmitted, so there is a chance that her interest in being a part of the practice development process will wane. In order to recruit more parents to work with the ward team on developing practice, Husna has made a display about the development of child and family-centred care for the ward notice board, including an invitation for parents to become a part of the process. She also asks parents who she thinks may be interested if they would like to participate. At the moment, two mothers are considering this.

The practicalities needed to sustain developments in practice

The people factors that are likely to influence how well the child and family-centred approach to care is maintained are key considerations for Husna. However, the resources, both financial and practical, that will enable this approach to be sustained long term are equally important (Hagedorn et al. 2006, Virani et al. 2009). This includes the time for staff to attend reflective sessions and funding for a facilitator's work remaining available. A part of

Husna showcasing specific examples of improvements that have resulted from the new approach to care is to illustrate value for money, and why the continued investment of time and resources is worthwhile.

As identified in Chapter 8, it is important to have managerial buy-in to practice development initiatives (McCormack et al. 2007). While the ward manager did not want to lead the process of developing child and family-centred care, he has always been committed to it. Yet Husna is aware that he is constantly faced with other competing operational goals, requirements and demands that have to be met (Carradice and Round 2004, Miller and Desmarais 2007). By working with him and understanding the competing demands he is juggling, she finds they are able to explore how short-term goals can be achieved without detracting from the central ethos of developing and maintaining child and family-centred care. This means that they continue to find solutions that satisfy the demands placed on her manager, without losing sight of the importance of child and family-centred processes.

As well as the resources needed to sustain the new ethos of care on a day-to-day basis, whether any ongoing education and training will be needed to achieve this requires consideration (Virani et al. 2009, Hall and Hord 2011). For Husna, this includes not just putting in place mechanisms to encourage those who are already working on the ward to remain committed to the ethos of child and family-centred care, but to enable those who join the team to adopt it. She has therefore developed a session for the new staff induction programme, which includes:

* how the ward regards child and family-centred care
* what the cultural expectation of staff is in this respect
* an introduction to reflective and high challenge/high support approaches to working.

New staff are also given specific support in these processes over their first three months in post. Husna sees this as vital to sustaining person-centred care because, unless its ethos and processes become embedded in new staff, as people come and go, it will eventually be lost. She also considers it important to highlight when they recruit staff that the ward uses this approach, so that those who take up posts are prepared for, and willing to engage in, this way of working.

Practice pointer 10.9

Sustaining a person-centred culture needs ongoing:

* resources
* time
* managerial buy-in
* preparation of new staff.

Activity 10.5

Identify a development in practice you know about that was not sustained (this may be the example used in Activity 10.1). Were resources an issue in this innovation not being sustained over time?

Keeping people informed

Keeping people informed of what is happening, as well as gaining and receiving feedback from those involved in the new way of working are vital in any change in practice. Effective and open communication is also a key part of the ethos underpinning practice development methodology (Dewing 2010). Husna is aware that, initially, this was a central part of the initiative and that as things progress, it needs to remain so. This includes her listening attentively to what people say, identifying positive events or influences, any problems or challenges that arise, and picking up on any undercurrents of disengagement or opposition that might be going on behind the scenes (Giangreco and Peccei 2005, Hall and Hord 2011). Maintaining open communication, listening to others and receiving challenging as well as positive feedback non-defensively are all things Husna considers important in terms of her continuing to role model what is expected in person-centred practice.

She also wants to be seen to collaborate with others in finding solutions to problems or challenges and progress in resolving difficulties being evident (Reed and Turner 2005, Hall and Hord 2011). To achieve this, she encourages those who have had difficulties and resolved them (or not) to share these in reflective group sessions so that they, as well as successes and positive developments, are seen to be transparently reported on and explored.

Keeping everyone informed of what is happening, seeking their views and feedback and being seen to act on these all indicate that people's opinions and feelings still matter (Giangreco and Peccei 2005, Hall and Hord 2011). Husna knows that if she is not seen to be engaging with the problems as well as the positives related to the new way of working, those who encounter difficulties or challenges may not think that they or their opinions and feelings are valued. This is likely to erode their enthusiasm for the initiative, and their experiences may also reduce other people's commitment (Cameron and Green 2009, Hall and Hord 2011). In addition, those who are opposed to the new developments will be able to use any lack of engagement with problems that Husna is thought to exhibit to encourage others to think that while developing more child and family-centred care may be good in theory, it is unworkable in practice. Husna has found that listening to what others say is also useful in terms of picking up on opposition that could slowly erode the ward's new approach to care, identifying unexpected problems or glitches, and demonstrating that the people involved, both staff and families, matter to her.

Practice pointer 10.10

Important aspects of sustaining enthusiasm for developing person-centred care are:

* keeping people informed
* giving feedback
* receiving and acting on feedback.

Activity 10.6

Identify a development in practice you know about that was not sustained (this may be the example used in Activity 10.1). Were people kept informed of progress, given, and invited to continue to give, feedback on the innovation?

Ongoing evaluation

A part of maintaining change is checking that the new way of working is still happening well after it has been introduced. Over the first year of the child and family-centred care initiative, Husna carried out formal evaluations that involved ascertaining the views of families and staff, and checking on how things worked over time, and with seasonal variations in workload. This enabled her to detect early warning signs of any movement away from more person-centred practice and, by feeding back from the evaluations, she was able to make the point that the new way of working was not forgotten. When things were going well, she could offer positive feedback and reinforcement to give people the incentive to keep going. On occasions when she felt things were slipping, she could provide reminders and explore what the problems with maintaining the initiative were.

Once the stimulus for change is gone, interest in it may diminish, and without reminders of why it was introduced, the problems that led to the innovation can be forgotten (Virani et al. 2009). Husna has therefore used the chance to feed back from evaluations as an opportunity to remind people where they have come from and where they are now, so that the benefits of the new way of working remain clear.

Husna does not want to overevaluate the development of child and family-centred care, but does want to keep it on people's agenda. She has decided that she will conduct a formal evaluation of what is happening every six months, compare this with the position six months previously, and with how things were at the outset of the initiative.

As well as formal evaluation mechanisms, Husna notes when any complaints or compliments about care provision are made, feeds them back to her colleagues, and includes them in the evaluation process. This not only gives her information about the way care is being provided and perceived, but also reminds people that, even when a formal evaluation is not taking place, she is aware of what is happening in relation to child and family-centred care.

Practice pointer 10.11

Ongoing evaluation:

- keeps the focus on person-centred care, despite competing priorities
- highlights the value of continuing to develop person-centred care
- reminds people of where practice has come from and what has already been achieved.

Activity 10.7

Identify a development in practice you know about that was not sustained (this may be the example used in Activity 10.1). Was there any ongoing evaluation of this initiative?

Planning ongoing developments

It has been suggested that change is more likely to be sustained if it is part of a cycle of events in which evaluation heralds further refinement and development of the new way of working, rather than being a linear event that ends with evaluation (Parkin 2009). Continually evaluating, tweaking and refining an innovation makes it difficult to go back to square one, because the change has become a part of something bigger, and square one no longer exists. By continuing the reflective activities and the high challenge/high support approach, Husna thinks it likely that people will continue to work in a more and more child and family-centred way, and that adopting any other approach will become less and less likely. She also makes a point of ensuring that practical and visible developments are noted, commented on and praised. People are also encouraged to note, and continue to note, their own development, so that the direction of travel remains clearly onwards and that an option of not using this approach seems distant and unlikely.

Summary

Husna thinks that sustaining the ethos of child and family-centred practice is as important as, and needs to be given equal attention to, its initial development. The greatest risk to any development in practice, including the development of a person-centred culture, is that people will slowly stop focusing on it, gradually make less effort to sustain it and it will eventually cease to exist. The efforts made to begin the process of developing person-centred practice therefore need to be followed by equal efforts to sustain such developments. These include processes, resources and leadership, succession planning, as well as mechanisms to prevent those who do not support the new way of working from eroding other people's participation. A further part of sustaining developments in practice is to continue to showcase and celebrate successes, including publicizing these within and outside the organization concerned.

Case scenario

Magda works on a medical ward specializing in the care of older people. Three years ago she was involved in leading an initiative aimed at developing more person-centred care on the ward. This included individuals engaging in reflective activities with a facilitator, group reflective sessions, and high challenge/high support mechanisms being used. The initiative involved nursing and medical staff, occupational therapists and physiotherapists, and the general feeling among the ward team was that practice had developed positively. However, they have recently realized that the person-centred culture they worked so hard to achieve is no longer prevalent, and Magda is considering why its initial successful development was not sustained.

Did competing priorities or new innovations and demands contribute to person-centred care not being sustained?

There is no one thing Magda can identify as displacing person-centred care, but the ward has frequently had to adopt new policies and protocols, and create and fulfil new roles and responsibilities, which have taken people's time, attention and energy. These factors, alongside a constantly heavy workload and the opening of four new beds, made it likely that other priorities slowly eroded people's focus on developing person-centred care. Over time, more and more reflective sessions were cancelled because of other meetings or workloads, and the established mechanisms of high challenge/high support faded out, ostensibly because people became too busy to sustain them. However, by looking at the rotas and dependency levels, Magda found that the workloads and staffing ratios did not change, it was more that the priority afforded to these activities receded over time. Having a high level of multidisciplinary involvement was a positive part of the process and contributed to the success of the initiative. Nevertheless, it meant that the competing priorities placed on every discipline involved affected the maintenance of the processes required to sustain person-centred care.

Were there any people on Magda's ward who never really supported the inno-vation in question? Did their influence increase or decrease over time?

Three or four staff members on Magda's ward initially opposed the idea of developing a more person-centred approach to care. They never engaged with it, but as other people became enthused by the idea, saw its positive outcomes and the idea gained momentum, their opposition seemed to fade away. However, they were probably a residual small, but significant force who chipped away at the success of person-centred care. Magda is sure that as new challenges and demands on people's time came along, those who opposed the new ethos of working would have encouraged people to prioritize other things. As more events related to developing person-centred care were missed, the overall force driving it would have diminished, and the significance of the views and actions of those who opposed it became proportionally greater.

Were there likely to have been any losses associated with this development that developed, increased, or became more apparent over time?

Magda cannot identify any particular new losses related to person-centred care that would have accrued over time. However, those who opposed the idea of becoming more person centred were initially quite open about this, and stated clearly that it would be one of those initiatives that was talked about, given a lot of time and attention, but would never get anywhere. Over time, as things appeared to progress, their sense of loss might have increased in terms of feeling more loss of the security of their established practice as more people adopted the new way of working. In addition, they might have begun to feel loss related to being wrong about their assumption that person-centred care would be a passing whim. These factors might have made them more determined to grasp the chance to contribute to its downfall as time went by.

Did the way in which leaders were developed influence person-centred care not being sustained?

Magda led the development of person-centred practice. It was never her intention to be the only or long-term leader of the process, but no one else was particularly keen to take on a lead role. One person agreed to do so, but subsequently become involved in developing a new care pathway for patients' discharge home, and did not feel able to take on both roles. As a result, when Magda was on her days off or annual leave, reflective sessions began to be missed because of other demands and no one else thought it was their place to insist on them. On reflection, Magda thought that one reason for the downfall of person-centred care was that it was ultimately seen as her responsibility, and not a shared initiative.

Were resources an issue in person-centred care not being sustained over time?

The key resources required to develop person-centred care on Magda's ward were:

- time for the staff to meet together and reflect
- payment for a facilitator for reflective sessions
- a location to meet in.

After a year or so, the facilitator's sessions decreased in number as intended, and eventually stopped, because the idea was for the processes of working in a person-centred way to become a core part of the ward team's work. However, Magda is not sure that the ward team truly developed the skills or confidence to sustain these processes. This, along with competing priorities and a lack of alternative leadership when she was not there, probably contributed to the development being eroded. Although there is a perception that the ward became too busy for person-centred care to be sustained, looking at the evidence from rotas and dependency levels, Magda thinks that priority and a lack of people to champion person-centred care in her absence, not time per se, was the issue.

Were people kept informed of progress, given, and invited to continue to give, feedback on person-centred care?

Magda was initially diligent about seeking feedback on how people were finding the process and outcomes of a more person-centred approach to care, and reported frequently on how things were going. Over time, though, and as reflective sessions dwindled, her seeking and giving of feedback became less frequent. In the early stages of developing person-centred care, achievements and anecdotes illustrating the positive aspects of this approach to care were reported in the trust newsletter, and the ward team published an article about their experiences. However, the celebration and showcasing of positive outcomes diminished over time, and at this point was no longer visible.

Was there any ongoing evaluation of person-centred care?

Magda carried out an evaluation of the development of person-centred care a year after the process began. This included individuals' perspectives of care, the processes being used, what worked well, what did not, and why this seemed to be the case. However, no further formal evaluations were conducted, which could have contributed to people gradually letting person-centred care fall off their radar.

Additional resources

www.institute.nhs.uk/documents/Useful%20Templates/P_LEAD_SI_POSTERS_
JAN22.pdf
*Provides information on the role of leadership in sustaining improvements in
healthcare.*

www.mckinsey.com/app_media/reports/financial_services/mcklean_winning.pdf
An article about sustaining change.

Sharing the Outcomes of Person-centred Practice Development

11

Chapter overview

- Developing person-centred practice is likely to generate information other people who want to develop practice in a similar way would find useful.
- Sharing information about developing person-centred practice locally is important, but it can also be valuable to share nationally and internationally through journals, publications and networking opportunities.
- Involving patients in the process of disseminating information about developments in practice is a key part of integrating them into the practice development process.

The community nursing team that Lucy works in has been involved in using the principles of practice development methodology to work towards a more person-centred approach to care. Lucy took a lead role in this process. Most people in the team wanted to try to work in this way, but the nature of their work and the makeup of the team (there are a number of part-time staff, some of whom only work one or two days a week) created some challenges. Finding time to meet together, and with a facilitator, was quite difficult, and one member of staff went on long-term sick leave soon after the process began, which left the team quite stretched for staff. They had several attempts at organizing times for discussions and reflective groups, and at one stage considered leaving the idea of developing more person-centred practice until their staffing levels were better. However, they decided against this, and eventually found a way of setting up reflective discussions and critical companionship that worked for them.

The team's journey to developing more person-centred care has been difficult, with a number of setbacks. However, a year on, they feel that they have made real progress, and the majority of them consider that their job satisfaction, as well as the quality of care patients experience, has improved. This view has been confirmed by feedback from patients.

Lucy thought that the team's journey to developing practice, and what they have achieved, should be publicized. Although their practice development activities are small scale and specific to them, they have generated information about the benefits, challenges and outcomes of developing person-centred practice that could be useful for other practitioners (Sheehan and Hayles 2006). Lucy's team have information on the way in which they used practice development methodology to develop person-centred care, but also on how they managed the practical process of achieving this, despite considerable challenges. This will almost certainly be useful for other teams to hear about, perhaps especially community nursing teams, who face similar staffing and workload issues. Lucy and her team are therefore now in the process of sharing their experiences of developing more person-centred practice.

Practice pointer 11.1

Sharing experiences of developing practice is important because:

- ideas for improving practice become known
- tips and techniques about what worked well can be shared
- challenges can be highlighted
- what did not work well can be identified.

Sharing locally

Those who have devoted time and effort to doing something should receive feedback on it, as a matter of courtesy, and because they need to know what has worked well, what has not, why this is thought to be the case, and what the next steps and future plans are. In addition, as Chapter 10 identified, keeping people informed of the outcomes of developments in practice serves as a reminder that the innovation is ongoing, and can encourage people to continue to input into it (Skinner 2004).

Although it is natural to think that the people know the outcomes of developments in practice they are involved in, this may not always be the case. Lucy realized that not everyone in the team would necessarily know the full extent of the outcomes of developing a more person-centred approach to care, or the plans for the continuation of this process. While everyone on the team attended reflective sessions, they did not all attend every one, and some people, especially those working part time, could easily miss information and updates on what colleagues were doing. This led Lucy to consider whether a more formal feedback mechanism within her team would be useful. She asked the team if they would be willing to contribute short statements or illustrations about how their work had developed, which she could make into a display in their office to celebrate how their practice had developed and how they had addressed the challenges they had faced. As well as encouraging all the team members, Lucy thought that displaying this information would enable visitors to the office to see what they had done and with what effect.

Lucy is also aware that many of the staff do not visit the office regularly, or only come in for short times. So, she is considering the best way to have the information on the display boards available for people who mainly work on the move. The options she has come up with are email updates, or creating an electronic notice board or forum where people can post and discuss what they are doing. She is unsure which, if any, of these options will be preferable, and does not know how to create an electronic notice board or forum. She has decided to discuss this with the team, so that they can create something accessible, but useful, rather than an electronic burden. If they decide on an electronic notice board or forum, she will be able to liaise with the organization's ICT department and seek guidance on how this would work.

Activity 11.1

List ways in which you might share a development in practice you have been involved in locally. How would you involve patients in this process?

Practice pointer 11.2

Sharing the outcomes of developing practice locally can:

- showcase everyone's hard work
- encourage ongoing participation
- provide colleagues with ideas and information about developments.

Publicizing your work outside your workplace

As well as feeding back to those involved in the new approach to work, Lucy and her team aim to share their practice development activities outside their immediate workplace. When they began their practice development journey, Lucy found plenty of information on the means they might use to develop person-centred practice, for example reflection, facilitation and critical companionship. However, it was much harder to find information about addressing the practical challenges of instigating these processes, such as rotas, staffing, how to find a facilitator, and how to decide if they were achieving the right balance between high challenge and high support. It would have been useful for them to have been able to read an example of how another team had approached this type of innovation, and hear in practical terms about what worked and what did not. The key issue, Lucy has realized, is not so much whether her team's experiences are extensive enough to merit sharing, but whether they can pull out the key issues that would matter to people who are trying to introduce something similar. This is likely to include explaining what they did and why they did it, and why what worked and what did not work.

Publicizing the team's work will also raise their profile, and although this is something of a secondary concern to them, it will be an additional bonus. Two approaches to getting information about what they have done into the public domain are written publications and conference presentations. The first thing that Lucy's team looked into was a written publication.

Practice pointer 11.3

Disseminating information about developments in practice includes deciding:

- who to tell
- what aspects of the developments to share
- how to share this information.

Publications

The first step for Lucy's team was to decide what aspects of their work they wanted to share and who they wanted to tell about their work. They concluded they wanted to share:

- the practical challenges that developing person-centred practice had posed for them
- how they overcame these
- the processes they used
- the benefits derived from the development of person-centred care.

Essentially, they decided to write a case study of the first year of their journey to developing person-centred practice.

The team wanted to aim their message at practitioners, but also had to think about exactly who within that broad category they would target, for example practitioners generally, those in a specific area, those from one profession or from more than one profession (Happell 2008, Price 2010). Lucy's team wanted to let other nurses working in the community know about their practice development activities, because they thought their experiences would be most pertinent to this group. So, they looked for journals aimed at community practitioners by searching in:

- www.mdlinx.com/nursing/journals.cfm
- www.rcn.org.uk/development/research_and_innovation/kt/dissemination/publish.

Having identified journals that might be suitable, Lucy looked at their websites to get the information for authors that described:

- the target audience for the journal
- what types of article they published
- how the manuscript should be presented
- how many words an article should have.

Having narrowed the list down to two journals, she looked at a recent edition of each journal to see what general tone and approach they used, and whether this matched what the team wanted to present. She thought they needed to be able to write enough to give a good overview of the team's work, but also to focus on what practitioners who were trying similar innovations might benefit from knowing. Lucy therefore looked for a journal that allowed at least 2,500 words for articles, and eventually selected one focused on community nursing that took articles up to 2,500 words long and was particularly interested in innovations in practice. This seemed the best option for what she and her team wanted to write about.

The journal Lucy selected was described as being 'peer reviewed'. This meant that an expert or experts in the field of practice that the article related to would assess the quality of the manuscript. These reviewers would decide whether the manuscript should be accepted as it was, with revisions made, or whether it lacked the essential quality requirements for publication. They might also decide that while it was of good quality, it was not suitable for this particular journal and recommend that it be submitted elsewhere. The journal in question stated that it used a 'double-blind peer review process', meaning that the writers' and reviewers' identities would not be disclosed to each other. Another way in which peer review can be managed is by 'open peer review', where the reviewers' and writers' identities are disclosed to one another. Although Lucy had not intentionally sought out a peer reviewed journal, she recognized that the scrutiny of peer review would mean that the journal was more highly regarded, as it provided some assurance that the articles in it were of good quality.

> **Practice pointer 11.4**
>
> Things to consider in planning an article:
>
> - the journal's target audience
> - the types of article the journal publishes
> - how many words an article should contain
> - the usual layout of articles.

Lucy and three key colleagues wrote the article together, but also acknowledged the rest of the nursing team, the patient representatives, and their facilitator and manager who were instrumental in the success of the innovation. As Lucy took the lead on the project and did most of the writing, she was named as the first author.

> **Activity 11.2**
>
> In relation to a development in practice you have been involved in:
>
> - Identify a journal you could write an article for.
> - Consider how you would include patients in the publication process.
> - Plan what you would include in your article.

Conferences

As well as writing for publication, Lucy and her colleagues have looked at conferences as an option for telling others about their work. Again, they had to decide what aspect of their work they wanted to focus on and for what audience.

Using conference listing websites, such as

- http://sites.google.com/site/consumerconferencesevents/medical-conferences-2011-2012-2013-2014-listings-by-specialism/nursing-care-conferences-congresses-2011-2012-2013-2014-us-uk-europe-asia-world
- www.rcn.org.uk/newsevents/events
- www.conferencealerts.com/topic-listing?topic=Nursing

they found numerous conferences targeting different audiences and with different focuses. The team also routinely receive various notifications about conferences. From these sources, they collated a list of four conferences they were interested in. One was a conference about practice development, two focused on community nursing and one was a more general nursing conference.

The team have decided that although they ideally want to keep their focus on the community aspect of their work, they are also interested in sharing the practicalities of using practice development methodology. They think that a particular contribution they can make is to highlight the practical challenges they have faced in developing practice, and the way they manage reflective sessions and use critical companionship. While avoiding repeating what they have said in their written paper, they want to feed back on the process of developing practice from a practical perspective. This is the thing they found hardest to find information on, and therefore a gap they feel they could usefully contribute to filling. They have decided to aim to present at the practice development conference, so that they can engage with a wider audience than just community nurses, and one that is primarily interested in developing practice.

The conference the team have selected gives a choice of applying to do a poster presentation or concurrent oral presentation. Lucy's team think that both options would be useful, but have decided to submit an abstract for a concurrent oral presentation, based on their experiences of the practicalities of using practice development methodology.

Activity 11.3

In relation to a development in practice you have been involved in:

- Look for a conference you could present this at.
- Consider how you would involve patients in the conference presentation process.
- List the things you would include in your conference presentation.

Partnership with patients

The central tenet of practice development methodology is that it is person centred. As such, the people who are most concerned in developments, patients, should play a central part in it. Lucy's team wanted to include patients in the process of developing person-centred practice from the outset, but found this difficult to achieve. As Chapter 5 identified, this can be a challenge in any practice development initiative. They initially asked for patient representatives to join them in the reflective sessions they held, but no patients expressed an interest. This might have been because of the challenges of timing, particularly as they were already struggling to organize reflective activities for staff, and it is possible that many patients were unable to attend at the times and venues offered. Because they were aware of a lack of patient input into the process, the team gave a major focus to how patients felt about their care in the evaluations of the practice development initiative. They also used the evaluation process to reiterate the invitation for patients to join the reflective activities, so that the team could benefit from understanding their perspectives. At this point, two people volunteered.

Involving patients in the dissemination of research findings is a logical part of them being partners in the research process (Cotterell et al. 2010). This principle applies equally to practice development activities, and therefore Lucy's team have considered how they can include their patient representatives in dissemination activities. They invited the two patient representatives to join them in preparing the paper for publication. Both felt that, having not been involved from the outset, they did not want to be a part of the writing, but agreed to proofread the paper and were acknowledged for this.

For the conference presentation, Lucy's team have asked whether the patient representatives would like to be a part of this, and share their experiences of the new way of working. One is happy to talk about what he has seen change and how he is now involved in the process of continuing to develop practice.

Practice pointer 11.5

Patients should be included in disseminating information about developing person-centred practice in a way that:

* matches their inclusion in the process
* is meaningful, and not tokenistic
* they feel comfortable with.

Networking

The traditional ways of disseminating information about innovations in practice have been local, national and international sharing via conferences and publications. However, it is becoming more common to also share information via a variety of electronic media and networks. Networks, be they electronic or otherwise, can be a useful and prompt way of sharing what works and what does not (McGeehan et al. 2009). In Lucy's team's case, formal and informal networks seem likely to be a valuable means of sharing their experiences directly with other practitioners.

There are a huge variety of networks available, some of which have been conducted via newsletters and meetings for many years. For example, Lucy is a member of a community nurses forum and can contribute to their newsletter and meetings. They also have an electronic forum where she can share information about what her team have achieved. Lucy has not used professional electronic networks before, and thinks that this forum may be a useful starting point for her. She is aware that sharing information electronically has to be approached with a degree of caution, and requires knowledge of whom she is sharing with, how secure the information is, and whether there is any risk of individual practitioners or patients being identified without their consent (Cann 2011). She feels that by using a network that is moderated by a group she is familiar with, and part of a professional organization, any inadvertent errors in how she shares and what she shares will be noted and addressed, and the information she divulges will be available to a secure and limited audience.

Other ways of sharing ideas are social media, such as Twitter, Facebook or blogging. There are pros and cons to using social media, but it can be a useful way of gaining and disseminating information, and makes information easily and rapidly available (Cann 2011, Rowlands et al. 2011). Social media can also allow those seeking and sharing information to discuss it, ask questions, and explore how things might work in particular settings (Cann 2011). Lucy is interested in this idea, but has never used Twitter, only uses Facebook for personal contacts, and has no experience of blogging. However, other members of her team are more adept at using social media than she is, and have agreed to look at networking and social media options. Lucy has also sought professional guidance on the issue, and looked into whether anyone in the organization's ICT and marketing departments can help and advise them on how best and safely to use social media to share their work.

Activity 11.4

Identify some networks where you might share information about an innovation in practice.

Practice pointer 11.6

Networking can be an effective and prompt way of sharing the process and outcomes of developing practice. This can include:

- meetings
- forums – electronic and face to face
- email lists
- discussion boards
- electronic social media.

While Lucy thinks that sharing and discussing what they had been involved in through networks will be useful, she also wants to avoid spending so much time on dissemination activities that the team become distracted from their ongoing work in developing person-centred care. The team have therefore decided that their journal article, conference presentation and the community nurses forum will be their key areas of dissemination for the time being.

Letting people know what doesn't work and why

Although disseminating information about developments in practice is often discussed in relation to talking about successes, it is equally useful to share what did not work and what was a struggle. If another team is planning a similar innovation to Lucy's team's, it will be useful for them to know about what is likely to work in practice, what is less likely to, and what may cause problems with, or improve the implementation of, person-centred working. This may prevent them from falling into known pitfalls, or embarking on a route that has a limited chance of success. Lucy thinks it is important for her team to share information about the way long-term sick leave and having several part-time staff impacted on their planning and implementation of reflective groups and critical companionship. She also believes that the questions they encountered over whether they were achieving the right balance between challenging each other and being supportive will be helpful for other teams to hear about.

A key issue the team struggled with is how to meaningfully integrate patients into the process of developing practice. Lucy thinks that in future they may be able to consider a whole article or presentation about how they approached this, including what helped and hindered them, and the assumptions, both correct and fallacious, they made. Although this is the area of their practice development activities she thinks was the least well managed, she also believes that it may be a valuable area for others to learn from, which will help them to avoid the pitfalls she and her team have experienced.

Summary

Lucy thinks that sharing the outcomes of her team's practice development activities may prove valuable, in terms of letting other people know what worked, what did not, and providing opportunities to share and learn from each other. The team plan to share their experiences with local, national and potentially international audiences through posters, publications, conference presentations, and electronic and social media. Each approach has benefits and challenges, and a key point for Lucy and her team has been to identify who the information is to be shared with and for what purpose. Including patients in the dissemination process is also important to them, so that their perspectives are represented, and their inclusion in practice development activities spans the whole process.

Case scenario

Jason was involved in leading a practice development initiative on the orthopaedic ward he works on. When the ward began the process of developing practice, their work was very task focused and centred on fairly rigid routines. However, over time, they have moved to being much more centred on the individual needs of people on the ward. They are now in the process of sharing the practicalities and challenges, as well as rewards and benefits, of this approach to care.

Jason and his team are sharing their practice development work locally, and involving patients in this process

Jason and his team have made a poster about their practice development journey to display on the ward notice board. This highlights the work that has been done and what has been achieved. They think this provides useful information and reminders for staff on where they came from and where they hope they are going. It also allows patients, visitors, people from other wards or departments, managers and external agencies to see their vision, achievements and what they aspire to. Jason has arranged for a copy of this poster to be placed on the hospital intranet to showcase their work.

Involving patients and relatives was a key part of developments in practice on the orthopaedic ward. Three patients volunteered to be involved in the process, and have contributed to making the poster.

Jason and his team identified a journal they could write an article for, decided how they would include patients in the writing process and planned what they would include in their article

Jason and his team decided to write an article for a general nursing journal. They thought that the processes they had gone through and the lessons they had learned would be beneficial to nurses working in any area, not just on orthopaedic wards. They searched for journals they could write for, and found one that took articles of up to 3,000 words and accepted papers that included research, innovations in practice and clinical articles.

The patients who were a part of the practice development process were involved in planning the article. One person wanted to contribute a section focused on patient involvement, while the other two were not very keen to write, but were happy to proofread the article before submission.

The key messages the team wanted to share were about the initial part of the practice development journey, because this was the most challenging part for them. They felt that, at a later stage, they could write another article about sustaining the process longer term. They planned their article as follows:

- Introduction: why the ward decided to develop practice to be more person centred (300 words)

- The principles of practice development methodology (300 words)
- The people in person-centred care: staff, managers, patients, relatives (250 words)
- Involving patients: who and how (350 words)
- The process:
  - personal and one-to-one reflection
  - reflective groups
  - high challenge/high support mechanisms (700 words)
- Challenges of implementing person-centred care (300 words)
- Initial evaluation: benefits and ongoing challenges (600 words)
- Conclusions and ongoing work (200 words).

Jason and his team looked for a conference they could present at, decided how they would include patients in this process and listed the things they would include in their conference presentation

Jason's team decided they would like to use a conference presentation to showcase the positive outcomes that using person-centred care had brought for staff and patients. They chose to submit an abstract to present a concurrent session at an orthopaedic nursing conference. They could have selected a general nursing conference, but thought some of the issues might be particularly pertinent to orthopaedic nursing, especially patients' perspectives.

Jason asked the patient representatives if they would participate in the conference presentation. They were keen to be involved, although one was uncertain they would be able to attend, alongside other commitments. However, they agreed that at least one of them would attend and share their experiences. Jason explained that, as yet, funding for anyone, including staff, was uncertain, but that he was looking to secure payment for all the conference places, although travel might need to be paid for by individuals.

The presentation allowed Jason and his team 20 minutes to present and 5 minutes for questions. They planned to present a brief overview of the theory and background to developing person-centred practice and the processes involved. Their main focus would be on showing how staff and patients had benefitted from the developments in practice. Their plan was as follows:

- Introduction: 4 minutes
- Patient perspectives: 7 minutes
- Staff perspectives: 7 minutes
- Conclusions: 2 minutes
- Questions and discussion: 5 minutes.

Networks where Jason and his team could share information about the development of person-centred practice

Jason and some of his colleagues belong to an orthopaedic nurses forum, and plan to share information on their practice development activities in meetings and via the group's email list. Jason has also discovered that the hospital has a Twitter account on which they have agreed to highlight Jason's ward's practice development activities.

One of the patients on the team asked about using her own Twitter account to spread the word about her involvement in the process of developing person-centred practice. She and Jason spoke to the hospital marketing team, and agreed what she would tweet on her own account.

Additional resources

Writing for publication
www.msu.edu/~budzynda/nursing/publishing.html
www.nurseauthoreditor.com/WritingforPublication2009.pdf
Provide information and guidance about writing for publication.

Presenting at conferences
http://nurse-practitioners-and-physician-assistants.advanceweb.com/Archives/
Article-Archives/Presenting-at-conferences-Rewarding-start-to-finish.aspx
Provides information and guidance on presenting at conferences.

Using social media
www.rin.ac.uk/our-work/communicating-and-disseminating-research/social-
media-guide-researchers
Discusses the benefits and challenges of using social media to share information.

Endpoints

The underpinning ethos of practice development methodology is person-centredness, and its aim is to develop person-centred cultures. It is a valuable approach to rigorously and systematically seeking to develop person-centred practice. Practice development methodology is influenced by the principles of critical social theory and critical realism, which consider how systems, structures, individual and group beliefs, values, norms and perceptions of reality contribute to what people do and their level of empowerment. As a result, it sees individuals and groups having the opportunity to explore how they currently work, what influences this, and how things could alter so that practice is more person centred as critical to enabling person-centred cultures to develop.

Practice development methodology does not focus on discrete aspects of practice, but aims to explore, in depth, personal and organizational cultures and how these can be developed in order to enhance the person-centredness of care. It can be useful for individuals and teams who are anywhere on the continuum of commencing the process of moving towards a person-centred culture to sustaining and refining an existing person-centred culture. To this end, the methods it uses focus on processes that can develop and hone people's skills in individual and group reflection, reflexivity and creative thinking. The intention is to create a culture in which there is a continuous process of people challenging, refining and developing the way they work, around the key issue of making this more person centred.

Personhood is the key focus of practice development methodology, and the processes it involves acknowledge the personhood of all those concerned – patients, their families and practitioners. These people should, therefore, work in partnership to develop person-centred practice, using dialogue in which their perspectives, values, priorities and constraints can be openly shared, and the humanity as well as citizenship of all parties acknowledged and respected.

Knowing people and developing practice based on this knowledge is the cornerstone of person-centred practice development. As a result, the evidence it uses focuses on understanding the beliefs, values, perceptions and priorities of patients, their relatives and practitioners, and the effect that their social and cultural situations have on them. However, knowledge gained from other sources, including research, audit, evaluation, expert opinion, case reports and clinical guidelines can also be useful in informing the development of person-centred care. The key issue is that the right type and quality of evidence is used for the right thing, and that the overall view, from all sources of evidence, is employed to give as full and in depth an understanding as possible to decision making. The intention of practice development methodology is to integrate evidence from practice and other types of evidence, and use these in ways that are applicable to particular practice situations in order to develop person-centred care.

Practice development methodology focuses on developing a more person-centred approach to care, rather than on changing particular elements of practice. Nonetheless, the principles of managing change can be useful in the process of encouraging individuals and teams to participate in the process of developing person-centred practice. This includes exploring those things that may contribute to individuals and groups not feeling able to engage in developments, such as:

- apathy
- fear of the losses they may encounter
- lack of confidence in their ability to participate in the process
- competing priorities
- time constraints.

In developing person-centred practice, the people factors that may act as driving or restraining forces for participation are key. The practical issues involved nonetheless also require consideration and planning in order for a person-centred way of working to be achievable.

Practice development methodology focuses on bottom-up, practitioner-owned changes in the way people work. Nevertheless, given the complexity of managing the people and processes involved, someone generally needs to take an overall lead in the process. For practice to develop in a person-centred way, it needs to be led in a way that matches a person-centred ethos. Approaches that are thought to achieve this include transformational and authentic leadership, which focus on leaders inspiring people to change the way they practise because of the intrinsic value of doing so, and not for the material rewards or punishments that will accrue because of it. Those who lead practice development initiatives may require preparation for, and support in, developing their roles; and for developments in practice to be sustained, succession planning for future leaders is a necessary consideration.

Developing person-centred practice is a continuous process, but formally evaluating its outcomes from time to time is important. This evaluation should incorporate the perspectives of all key stakeholders, and include not just whether or not practice has developed to be more person centred, but why this is so. The process of evaluating the outcomes of using practice development methodology needs to be consistent with its person-centred ethos, and the principles of realistic evaluation may provide a useful framework for achieving this. Realistic evaluation, like practice development methodology, acknowledges different perspectives and types of knowledge and the influence of these and the social and contextual situation in which events occur on the success or otherwise of innovations. It also recognizes the need for ongoing cycles of action, evaluation and further refining of developments in practice.

Developing person-centred practice is an ongoing process, and as well as initial developments, processes to sustain and extend these are a vital part of creating person-centred cultures. The greatest threat to a person-centred culture being sustained is it being slowly eroded by other priorities and demands. Measures that can be useful in preventing this include:

- linking new innovations and requirements to the ethos of person-centredness
- highlighting ongoing developments in person-centred care and their benefits
- understanding losses that may accrue and develop over time
- being aware of anyone who continues to oppose this way of working
- succession planning for leadership roles and patient participation
- securing continued resources and managerial buy-in
- preparing new staff for this approach
- continuing to provide but also seeking and acting on feedback about the processes and outcomes of person-centred practice development.

Engaging in the process of developing person-centred practice is likely to generate information that will be useful to other individuals or teams who are interested in developing practice in a similar way. Disseminating such information is an important part of enabling the overall quality of care within health services to improve, because it allows others to gain insights into what may or may not work for them. It may also guide those who are considering whether or not to seek to develop practice in this way to better understand the practicalities of how it can be achieved. Thus, sharing experiences of developing person-centred practice locally, but also nationally and internationally through journals, publications and networking opportunities, is valuable. Patients being a part of the process of disseminating information about person-centred practice development is a key element of integrating them into the process of developing practice, and enabling others to see how this can be achieved.

Developing person-centred practice is a process, not a product. Enabling people to develop the skills and mental space to question, refine and develop the way they approach practice takes time, effort and commitment, and produces results that, over time, are invaluable. However, these cannot be rushed, as they require people to genuinely engage in exploring their views and perspectives, and authentically questioning their own thinking. Practice development methodology is not intended to provide quick fixes for urgent problems, and one of the challenges of developing person-centred practice is to enable people to see the value of investing long term in this type of development. For care to become and, perhaps even more importantly, remain person centred, ongoing commitment to the processes that allow this to develop and flourish is required.

References

Albarran JW (2004) 'Creativity: an essential element of critical care nursing practice', *Nursing in Critical Care* 9, 2, 47–9.

Aleem IS, Jalal H, Aleem IS, Sheikh AA and Bhandari M (2009) 'Clinical decision analysis: incorporating the evidence with patient preferences', *Patient Preference and Adherence* 3, 21–4.

Allan E (2007) 'Change management for school nurses in Scotland', *Nursing Standard* 21, 42, 35–9.

Armstrong N, Herbert G, Aveling E-L, Dixon-Woods M and Martin G (2013) 'Optimizing patient involvement in quality improvement', *Health Expectations* 16, 3, e36–47.

Astin F (2009) 'A beginner's guide to appraising a qualitative research paper', *British Journal of Cardiac Nursing* 4, 11, 530–3.

Atwal A and Jones M (2007) 'The importance of the multidisciplinary team', *British Journal of Healthcare Assistants* 19, 9, 425–8.

Austin J and Currie B (2003) 'Changing organizations for a knowledge economy: the theory and practice of change management', *Journal of Facilities Management* 2, 3, 229–43.

Avolio BJ, Walumbwa FO and Weber TJ (2009) 'Leadership: current theories, research, and future directions', *Annual Review of Psychology* 60, 1, 421–49.

Balasubramanian BA, Chase SM, Nutting PA, Cohen DJ, Strickland PA et al. (2010) 'Using Learning Teams for Reflective Adaptation (ULTRA): insights from a team-based change management strategy in primary care', *Annals of Family Medicine* 8, 5, 425–32.

Balls P (2009) 'Phenomenology in nursing research: methodology, interviewing and transcribing', *Nursing Times* 105, 32/3, 30–3.

Barnum BS (2010) 'Should spiritual care be a function of nursing practice?', pp. 119–27, in Barnum BS *Spirituality in Nursing: The Challenges of Complexity* (3rd edn). (New York: Springer).

Barnett-Page E and Thomas J (2009) 'Methods for the synthesis of qualitative research: a critical review', BMC Medical Research Methodology, 9, 59, 1–11.

Bartlett R and O'Connor D (2007) 'From personhood to citizenship: broadening the lens for dementia practice and research', *Journal of Aging Studies* 21, 2, 107–18.

Beauchamp TL and Childress JF (2008) *Principles of Biomedical Ethics* (6th edn). (Oxford: Oxford University Press).

Beresford P (2010) 'Public partnerships, governance and user involvement: a service user perspective', *International Journal of Consumer Studies* 34, 5, 495–502.

Bergin M, Wells JS and Owen S (2008) 'Critical realism: a philosophical framework for the study of gender and mental health', *Nursing Philosophy* 9, 169–79.

Bevan JL, Senn-Reeves JN, Inventor BR, Greiner SM, Mayer KM et al. (2012) 'Critical social theory approach to disclosure of genomic incidental findings', *Nursing Ethics* 19, 6, 819–28.

Blamey A and Mackenzie M (2007) 'Theories of change and realistic evaluation: peas in a pod or apples and oranges?', *Evaluation* 13, 4, 439–55.

Boomer CA and McCormack B (2010) 'Creating the conditions for growth: a collaborative practice development programme for clinical nurse leaders', *Journal of Nursing Management* 18, 6, 633–44.

Borg M, Karlsson B and Kim HS (2009) 'User involvement in community mental health services-principles and practices', *Journal of Psychiatric and Mental Health Nursing* 16, 3, 285–92.

Borg M, Karlsson B, Kim HS and McCormack B (2012) 'Opening up for many voices in knowledge construction', *Forum: Qualitative Social Research* 13, 1, Art. 1, http://nbn-resolving.de/urn:nbn:de:0114-fqs120117, accessed 13/3/14.

Bradshaw PL (2008) 'Service user involvement in the NHS in England: genuine user participation or a dogma-driven folly?', *Journal of Nursing Management* 16, 6, 673–81.

Branson C (2007) 'Effects of structured self-reflection on the development of authentic leadership practices among Queensland primary school principals', *Educational Management Administration and Leadership* 35, 2, 225–46.

Bray L, Brown J, Prescott T and Moen C (2009) 'Exploring the process of becoming and working as a practice development unit', *Practice Development in Health Care* 8, 4, 186–99.

Braye S and Preston-Shoot M (2005) 'Emerging from out of the shadows? Service user and carer involvement in systematic reviews', *Evidence and Policy* 1, 2, 173–93.

Brown D and McCormack BG (2011) 'Developing the practice context to enable more effective pain management with older people: an action research approach', *Implementation Science* 6, 9, 1–14.

Bryman A (2006) 'Integrating quantitative and qualitative research: How is it done?', *Qualitative Research* 6, 1, 97–113.

Buchanan D, Fitzgerald L, Ketley D, Gollop R, Jones JL et al. (2005) 'No going back: a review of the literature on sustaining organizational change', *International Journal of Management Reviews* 7, 3, 189–205.

Burla L, Knierim B, Barth J, Liewad K, Duetz M et al. (2008) 'From text to codings', *Nursing Research* 57, 2, 113–17.

Burton C (2004) *Understanding how Research is Presented* (London: Distance Learning Centre, South Bank University).

Busser D (2012) 'Delivering effective performance feedback', *Training and Development,* 66, 4, 32–4.

Cameron E and Green M (2009) *Making Sense of Change Management: A Complete Guide to the Models, Tools and Techniques of Organizational Change* (2nd edn). (London: Kogan Page).

Campos CJG and Turato ER (2009) 'Content analysis in studies using the clinical-qualitative method: application and perspectives', *Revista Latino-Americana de Enfermagem* 17, 2, 259–64.

Cann A (2011) Social media: a guide for researchers. Available at www.rin.ac.uk/social-media-guide, accessed 14/3/14.

Carradice A and Round D (2004) 'The reality of practice development for nurses working in an inpatient service for people with severe and enduring mental health problems', *Journal of Psychiatric and Mental Health Nursing* 11, 6, 731–7.

Carroll J and Quijada M (2004) 'Redirecting traditional professional values to support safety: changing organizational culture in healthcare', *Quality and Safety in Healthcare* 13, supplement ii, 16–21.

CASP (Critical Appraisal Skills Programme) (2010) Making sense of evidence about clinical effectiveness. Available at www.caspinternational.org/mod_product/uploads/CASP_Systematic_Review%20_Checklist_14.10.10.pdf, accessed 3/9/14.

Chan ZCY (2013) 'Exploring creativity and critical thinking in traditional and innovative problem-based learning groups', *Journal of Clinical Nursing* 22, 2298–307.

Chin H and Hamer S (2006) 'Enabling practice development: evaluation of a pilot programme to effect integrated and organic approaches to practice development', *Practice Development in Health Care* 5, 3, 126–44.

Chin R and Benne KD (1985) 'General strategies for effecting change in human systems', pp. 22–45, in Bennis WD, Benne KD and Chin R (eds) *The Planning of Change* (4th edn). (New York: Holt Rinehart & Winston).

Cloninger CR (2011) 'Person-centred integrative care', *Journal of Evaluation in Clinical Practice* 17, 2, 371–2.

Clough P and Nutbrown C (2012) *The Student's Guide to Methodology* (3rd edn). (London: Sage).

Comfort H (2010) *Practical Guide to Outcome Evaluation* (London: Jessica Kingsley).

Cork A (2005) 'A model for successful change management', *Nursing Standard* 19, 25, 40–2.

Cotterell P, Harlow G, Morris C, Beresford P, Hanley B et al. (2010) 'Service user involvement in cancer care: the impact on service users', *Health Expectations* 14, 2, 159–69.

Coughlan M, Cronin P and Ryan F (2007) 'Step by-step guide to critiquing research. Part 1: quantitative research', *British Journal of Nursing* 16, 11, 658–63.

CQC (Care Quality Commission) (2012) *The State of Health Care and Adult Social Care in England* (London: TSO).

Creswell JW (2003) *Research Design: Qualitative, Quantitative, and Mixed Methods Approaches* (2nd edn). (Thousand Oaks, CA: Sage).

Crombie IK and Davis HT (2009) *What is Meta-analysis?* (2nd edn). (Hayward Medical Communications), www.whatisseries.co.uk/whatis/pdfs/What_is_meta_analy.pdf, accessed 15/3/14.

Cruickshank J (2012) 'Positioning positivism, critical realism and social constructionism in the health sciences: a philosophical orientation', *Nursing Inquiry* 19, 1, 71–82.

Curry LA, Nembhard IM and Bradley EH (2009) 'Qualitative and mixed methods provide unique contributions to outcomes research', *Circulation* 119, 10, 1442–52.

Deeks JJ, Higgins JPT and Altman DG (2011) 'Analysing data and undertaking meta analyses', Chapter 9, in Higgins JT and Green S (eds) *Cochrane Handbook for Systematic Reviews of Interventions*, Version 5.1.0 (The Cochrane Collaboration), available from www.cochrane-handbook.org, accessed 14/3/14.

Dewing J, Brooks J and Ridaway L (2006) 'Research and review involving older people in practice development work: an evaluation of an intermediate care service and practice', *Practice Development in Health Care* 5, 3, 156–74.

Dewing J (2008) 'Becoming and being active learners and creating active learning workplaces: the value of active learning', pp. 273–94, in McCormack B, Manley K and Wilson V (eds) *International Practice Development in Nursing and Healthcare* (Oxford: Blackwell).

Dewing J (2010) 'Moments of movement: active learning and practice development', *Nurse Education in Practice* 10, 1, 22–6.

DH (Department of Health) (2012) *Health and Social Care Act* (London: DH).

DH (2013) *Compassion in Practice. Nursing, Midwifery and Care Staff: Our Vision and Strategy* (Leeds: NHS Commissioning Board).

Diaz del Campo P, Gracia J, Blasco JA and Andradas E (2011) 'A strategy for patient involvement in clinical practice guidelines: methodological approaches', *BMJ Quality and Safety in Healthcare* 20, 9, 779–84.

Diddams M and Chang GC (2012) 'Only human: exploring the nature of weakness in authentic leadership', *The Leadership Quarterly* 23, 3, 593–603.

Dixon-Woods M, Bonas S, Booth A, Jones DR, Miller T et al. (2006) 'How can systematic reviews incorporate qualitative research? A critical perspective', *Qualitative Research* 6, 1, 27–44.

Donnelly P and Kirk P (2010) 'How to … give effective feedback', *Education for Primary Care* 21, 4, 267–9.

Doody O and Doody CM (2012) 'Transformational leadership in nursing practice', *British Journal of Nursing* 21, 20, 1212–18.

Edvardsson D, Fetherstonhaugh D and Nay R (2010) 'Promoting a continuation of self and normality: person-centred care as described by people with dementia, their family members and aged care staff', *Journal of Clinical Nursing* 19, 17/18, 2611–18.

Erwin DG and Garman AN (2010) 'Resistance to organizational change: linking research and practice', *Leadership and Organizational Development Journal* 31, 1, 39–56.

Evans DH, Bacon RJ, Greer E, Stagg AM and Turton P (2013) 'Calling executives and clinicians to account: user involvement in commissioning cancer services', *Health Expectations* doi:10.1111/hex.12051.

Ferrance E (2000) *Action Research* (Providence, RI: Brown University).

Fielding C, Rooke D, Graham I and Keen S (2008) 'Reflections on a "virtual" practice development unit: changing practice through identity development', *Journal of Clinical Nursing* 17, 10, 1312–19.

Finset A (2011) 'Research on person-centred clinical care', *Journal of Evaluation in Clinical Practice* 17, 2, 384–6.

Francis R (2013) *Report of the Mid Staffordshire NHS Foundation Trust Public Inquiry* (London: TSO).

Freeman M and Vasconcelos EFS (2010) 'Critical social theory: core tenets, inherent issues', in M. Freeman (ed.) *Critical Social Theory and Evaluation Practice. New Directions for Evaluation*, 127, 7–19.

Fronda Y and Moriceau JL (2008) 'I am not your hero: change management and culture shocks in a public sector corporation', *Journal of Organizational Change Management* 21, 5, 589–609.

Garbarino S and Holland J (2009) *Quantitative and Qualitative Methods in Impact Evaluation and Measuring Results* (London: Governance and Social Development Resource Centre/Department for International Development).

Gardner WL, Avolio BJ, Luthans F, May DR and Walumbwa F (2005) '"Can you see the real me?" A self-based model of authentic leader and follower development', *The Leadership Quarterly* 16, 3, 343–72.

Giangreco A and Peccei R (2005) 'The nature and antecedents to middle manager resistance to change: evidence from an Italian context', *International Journal of Human Resource Management* 16, 10, 1812–29.

GMC (General Medical Council) (2013) *Good Medical Practice* (London: GMC).

Golden B (2006) 'Change: transforming healthcare organizations', *Healthcare Quarterly* 10, special issue, 10–19.

Goodman B (2008) 'Crunch the numbers', *Nursing Standard* 22, 29, 49.

Gopikrishna V (2010) 'A report on case reports', *Journal of Conservative Dentistry* 13, 4, 265–71.

Grol R and Grimshaw J (2003) 'From best evidence to best practice: effective implementation of change in a patients' care', *The Lancet* 362, 9391, 1225–30.

Habermas JT (1971) *Knowledge and Human Interests* (Boston, MA: Beacon Press).

Hagedorn H, Hogan M, Smith JL, Bowman C, Curran GM et al. (2006) 'Lessons learned about implementing research evidence into clinical practice', *Journal of General Internal Medicine* 21, S21–4.

Hahn DL (2009) 'Importance of evidence grading for guideline implementation: the example of asthma', *Annals of Family Medicine* 7, 4, 364–9.

Halcomb EJ, Andrew S and Brannen J (2009) 'Introduction to mixed methods research for nursing and the health sciences', pp. 3–12, in Andrews S and Halcomb EJ (eds) *Mixed Methods Research for Nursing and the Health Sciences* (Chichester: Wiley-Blackwell).

Hall GE and Hord SM (2011) *Implementing Change: Patterns, Principles and Potholes* (3rd edn). (London: Pearson).

Happell B (2008) 'Writing for publication: a practical guide', *Nursing Standard* 22, 28, 35–40.

Harvey G and Wensing M (2003) 'Methods for evaluation of small scale quality improvement projects', *Quality and Safety in Healthcare* 12, 210–14.

Harwood L and Clark AM (2012) 'Understanding health decisions using critical realism: home-dialysis decision-making during chronic kidney disease', *Nursing Inquiry* 19, 1, 29–38.

Haveri A (2008) 'Evaluation of change in local governance: the rhetorical wall and the politics of images', *Evaluation* 14, 2, 141–55.

HCPC (Health and Care Professions Council) (2012) *Your Duty as a Registrant: Your Guide to Our Standards for Continuing Professional Development* (London: HCPC).

Hemingway A and Cowdell F (2009) 'Perspectives in public health using practice development methodology to develop children's centre teams: ideas for the future', *Perspectives in Public Health* 129, 5, 234–8.

Hewitt-Taylor J (2011) *Using Research in Practice: It Sounds Good, But Will It Work?* (Basingstoke: Palgrave Macmillan).

Higgins A, McGuire G, Watts M, Creaner M, McCann E et al. (2011) 'Service user involvement in mental health practitioner education in Ireland', *Journal of Psychiatric and Mental Health Nursing* 18, 519–25.

Holma K and Kontinen T (2011) 'Realistic evaluation as an avenue to learning for development NGOs', *Evaluation* 17, 2, 181–92.

Holt DT, Armenakis AA, Harris SG and Field HS (2007) 'Toward a comprehensive definition of readiness for change: a review of research and instrumentation', *Research in Organizational Change and Development* 16, 289–336.

Hoole L and Morgan S (2010) '"It's only right that we get involved": service-user perspectives on involvement in learning disability services', *British Journal of Learning Disabilities* 39, 1, 5–10.

Hughes R (2008) 'Understanding audit: methods and application', *Nursing and Residential Care* 11, 2, 88–91.

Iles V and Cranfield S (2004) *Managing Change in the NHS. Developing Change Management Skills: A Resource for Health Care Professionals and Managers* (London: National Co-ordinating Centre for NHS Service Delivery and Organization, Research and Development).

Innes A, Macpherson S and McCabe L (2006) *Promoting Person-Centred Care at the Front Line* (York: Joseph Rowntree Foundation).

Jackson SF and Kolla G (2012) 'A new realistic evaluation analysis method: linked coding of context, mechanism, and outcome relationships', *American Journal of Evaluation* 33, 3, 339–49.

Jeyasingham M (2008) 'Cultural diversity and research: the use of realistic evaluation and the role of the nurse', *Journal of Research in Nursing* 13, 2, 83–5.

Johnson RB and Onwuegbuzie AJ (2004) 'Mixed methods research: a research paradigm whose time has come', *Educational Researcher* 33, 7, 14–26.

Jordan Z (2009) 'Magnet recognition and practice development: two journeys towards practice improvement in health care', *International Journal of Nursing Practice* 15, 6, 495–501.

Kearney MH (2005) 'Seeking the sound bite: reading and writing clinically useful qualitative research', *Journal of Obstetric, Gynecologic and Neonatal Nursing* 34, 4, 417.

Kempster S (2009) 'Observing the invisible: the development of leadership practice', *Journal of Management Development* 28, 5, 439–56.

King K and Kelly D (2011) 'Practice development in community nursing: opportunities and challenges', *Nursing Standard* 25, 30, 38–44.

Kirkley C, Bamford C, Poole M, Arksey H, Hughes J et al. (2011) 'The impact of organisational culture on the delivery of person-centred care in services providing respite care and short breaks for people with dementia', *Health and Social Care in the Community* 19, 4, 438–48.

Koch T (2006) 'Establishing rigour in qualitative research: the decision trail', *Journal of Advanced Nursing* 53,1, 91–100.

Kotter JP (1995) 'Leading change: why transformation efforts fail', *Harvard Business Review* 73, 2, 1–10.

Krueger G (2006) 'Meaning making in the aftermath of sudden infant death syndrome', *Nursing Inquiry* 13, 3, 163–71.

Kumar CR (2008) *Research Methodology* (New Delhi: APH Publishing).

Lapum J, Hamzavi N, Veljkovic K, Mohamed Z, Pettinato A et al. (2012) 'A performative and poetical narrative of critical social theory in nursing education: an ending and threshold of social justice', *Nursing Philosophy* 13, 27–45.

Larsen JA, Maundrill R, Morgan J and Mouland L (2005) 'Practice development facilitation: an integrated strategic and clinical approach', *Practice Development in Health Care* 4, 3,142–9.

Lee P (2006) 'Understanding and critiquing quantitative research papers', *Nursing Times* 102, 28, 28–30.

Lewin K (1951) *Field Theory in Social Science: Selected Theoretical Papers* (New York: Harper & Row).

Lhussier M, Carr SM and Robson A (2008) 'The potential contribution of realistic evaluation to small-scale community interventions', *Community Practitioner* 81, 9, 25–8.

LoBiondo-Wood G and Haber J (2005) *Nursing Research Methods and Critical Appraisal for Evidence-based Practice* (6th edn). (St Louis, MO: Mosby Elsevier).

Lothian JA (2005) 'Creating change and staying connected through collaboration', *Journal of Perinatal Education* 14, 4, 36–9.

Ludwick DA and Doucette J (2009) 'The implementation of operational processes for the Alberta Electronic Health Record: lessons from electronic medical record adoption in primary care', *Electronic Healthcare* 7, 4, 103–7.

McCabe D (2010) 'Taking the long view: a cultural analysis of memory as resisting and facilitating organizational change', *Journal of Organizational Change Management* 23, 3, 230–50.

McCance T, Slater P and McCormack B (2008) 'Using the caring dimensions inventory as an indicator of person-centred nursing', *Journal of Clinical Nursing* 18, 3, 409–17.

McCarthy B (2006) 'Translating person-centred care: a case study of preceptor nurses and their teaching practices in acute care areas', *Journal of Clinical Nursing* 15, 5, 629–38.

McCormack B (2003) 'A conceptual framework for person-centred practice with older people', *International Journal of Nursing Practice* 9, 3, 202–9.

McCormack B (2004) 'Person-centredness in gerontological nursing: an overview of the literature', *Journal of Clinical Nursing* 13, 3a, 31–8.

McCormack B (2006) 'Evidence-based practice and the potential for transformation', *Journal of Research in Nursing* 11, 2, 89–94.

McCormack B (2008) 'Practice development: "to be what we want to be"', *Journal of Clinical Nursing* 18, 2, 160–2.

McCormack B and McCance T (2006) 'Development of a framework for person-centred nursing', *Journal of Advanced Nursing* 56, 5, 472–9.

McCormack B and McCance T (2010) *Person-centred Nursing: Theory and Practice* (Chichester: Wiley-Blackwell).

McCormack B and Titchen A (2006) 'Critical creativity: melding, exploding, blending', *Educational Action Research* 14, 2, 239–66.

McCormack B, Manley K and Titchen A (2013) 'Introduction', pp. 1–17, in McCormack B, Manley K and Titchen A (eds) *Practice Development in Nursing and Healthcare* (2nd edn). (Chichester: Wiley Blackwell).

McCormack B, Karlsson B, Dewing J and Lerdal A (2010) 'Exploring person-centeredness: a qualitative meta-synthesis of four studies', *Scandinavian Journal of Caring Sciences* 24, 3, 620–34.

McCormack B, Roberts T, Meyer J, Morgan D and Boscart V (2012) 'Appreciating the "person" in long-term care', *International Journal of Older People Nursing* 7, 4, 284–94.

McCormack B, Wright J, Dewar B, Harvey G and Ballantine K (2007) 'A realist synthesis of evidence relating to practice development: recommendations', *Practice Development in Health Care* 6, 1, 76–80.

McCormack B, Dewar B, Wright J, Garbett R, Harvey G et al. (2006) *A Realist Synthesis of Evidence Relating to Practice Development*: Final Report to NHS Education for Scotland and NHS Quality Improvement Scotland (University of Ulster/NHS Education for Scotland/NHS Quality Improvement Scotland/University of Manchester Business School) Available at www. healthcareimprovementscotland.org/previous_resources/archived/pd_-_ evidence_synthisis.aspx, accessed 14/3/14.

McCormack B, Dewing J, Breslin L, Coyne-Nevin A, Kennedy K et al. (2009) 'Practice development: realising active learning for sustainable change', *Contemporary Nurse* 32, 1/2, 92–104.

McDonnell A, Wilson R and Goodacre S (2006) 'Evaluating and implementing new services', *British Medical Journal* 332, 7533, 109–12.

McGaughey J, Blackwood B, O'Halloran P, Trinder TJ and Porter S (2010) 'Realistic evaluation of early warning systems and the acute life-threatening events recognition and treatment training course for early recognition and management of deteriorating ward-based patients: research protocol', *Journal of Advanced Nursing* 66, 4, 923–32.

McGeehan B, Debbage S, Gilsenan I, Jennings A, Jennings C et al. (2009) 'Supporting clinical innovation: an organization-wide approach to practice-based development', *Practice Development in Health Care* 8, 1, 18–27.

McGilton KS, Heath H, Chu CH, Boström A-M, Mueller C et al. (2012) 'Moving the agenda forward: a person-centred framework in long-term care', *International Journal of Older People Nursing* 7, 4, 303–9.

McGrath JE and Johnson BA (2003) 'Methodology makes meaning: how both qualitative and quantitative paradigms shape evidence and its interpretation', pp. 31–8, in Camic PM, Rhodes JE and Yardley L (eds) *Qualitative Research in Psychology: Expanding Perspectives in Methodology and Design* (Washington DC: APA Books).

McKay R, McDonald R, Lie D and McGowan H (2012) 'Reclaiming the best of the biopsychosocial model of mental health care and "recovery" for older people through a "person-centred" approach', *Australasian Psychiatry: Bulletin of Royal Australian and New Zealand College of Psychiatrists* 20, 6, 492–5.

McKeown J, Clarke A, Ingleton C, Ryan T and Repper J (2010) 'The use of life story work with people with dementia to enhance person-centered care', *International Journal of Older People Nursing* 5, 2, 148–58.

McLean C (2011) 'Change and transition: what is the difference?', *British Journal of School Nursing* 6, 2, 78–81.

MacLeod R and McPherson KM (2007) 'Care and compassion: part of person-centred rehabilitation, inappropriate response or a forgotten art?', *Disability and Rehabilitation* 29, 20/1, 1589–95.

Macphee M and Suryaprakash N (2012) 'First-line nurse leaders' health-care change management initiatives', *Journal of Nursing Management* 20, 2, 249–59.

Manley K and McCormack B (2003) 'Practice development: purpose, methodology, facilitation and evaluation', *Nursing in Critical Care* 8, 1, 22–9.

Manley K and McCormack B (2004) 'Practice development, purpose, methodology, facilitation and evaluation', pp. 33–50, in McCormack B, Manley K and Garbett R (eds) *Practice Development in Nursing* (Chichester: Wiley-Blackwell).

Manley K and McCormack B (2008) 'Person-centred care', *Nursing Management* 15, 8, 12–13.

Manley K, Hills V and Marriot S (2011) 'Person-centred care: principle of nursing practice D', *Nursing Standard* 25, 31, 35–7.

Manley K, Titchen A and Hardy S (2009) 'Work-based learning in the context of contemporary health care education and practice: a concept analysis', *Practice Development in Health Care* 8, 2, 87–127.

Manley K, Titchen A and McCormack B (2013a) 'What is practice development and what are the starting points?', pp. 45–65, in McCormack B, Manley K and Titchen A (eds) *Practice Development in Nursing and Healthcare* (2nd edn). (Chichester: Wiley-Blackwell).

Manley K, Solman A and Jackson C (2013b) 'Working towards a culture of effectiveness in the workplace', pp. 146–68, in McCormack B, Manley K and Titchen A (eds) *Practice Development in Nursing and Healthcare* (2nd edn). (Chichester: Wiley-Blackwell).

May DR, Chan AY, Hodges TD and Avolio BJ (2003) 'Developing the moral component of authentic leadership', *Organizational Dynamics* 32, 3, 247–60.

Mertens DM (2005) *Research and Evaluation in Education and Psychology: Integrating Diversity with Quantitative, Qualitative and Mixed-Methods* (2nd edn). (Thousand Oaks, CA: Sage).

Miller D and Desmarais S (2007) 'Developing your talent to the next level: five best practices for leadership development', *Organization Development Journal* 25, 3, 37–43.

Moody RC and Pesut DJ (2006) 'The motivation to care: application and extension of motivation theory to professional nursing work', *Journal of Health Organization and Management* 20, 1, 15–48.

Moore M (2008) 'Appreciative inquiry: the why: the what? the how?', *Practice Development in Health Care* 7, 4, 214–20.

Newman C, Cashin A and Downie A (2009) 'An evaluation of nurse engagement in emancipatory practice development: the diary of a critical companion', *Practice Development in Health Care* 8, 2, 77–86.

NICE (National Institute for Health and Clinical Excellence) (2005) *Assessing Evidence and Recommendations in NICE Guidelines: Paper for SMT*, www.nice.org.uk/niceMedia/pdf/smt/251005item3.pdf, accessed 13/03/2014.

NICE (2007) *How to Change Practice* (London: NICE).

NICE (2009) *The Guidelines Manual* (London: NICE).

NMC (Nursing and Midwifery Council) (2008) *The Code: Standards of Conduct, Performance and Ethics for Nurses and Midwives* (London: NMC).

NPSA/NRES (National Patient Safety Agency/National Research Ethics Service) (2009) *Defining Research* (London: NPSA/NRES).

Nussbaum A and Dweck C (2008) 'Defensiveness versus remediation: self-theories and modes of self-esteem maintenance', *Personality and Social Psychology Bulletin* 34, 5, 599–612.

Oakland JS and Tanner SJ (2007) 'A new framework for managing change', *The TQM Magazine* 19, 6, 572–89.

O'Boyle-Duggan M and Gretch J (2012) 'Service user involvement in student selection', *Learning Disability Practice* 15, 4, 20–5.

Oliver C (2012) 'Critical realist grounded theory: a new approach for social work research', *British Journal of Social Work* 42, 2, 371–87.

Oxman AD and Flottorp S (2001) 'An overview of strategies to promote implementation of evidence-based health care', pp 101–19, in Silagy C and Haines A (eds) *Evidence-Based Practice in Primary Care* (2nd edn). (London: BMJ Books).

Paré G, Sicotte C, Poba-Nzaou P and Balouzakis G (2011) 'Clinicians' perceptions of organizational readiness for change in the context of clinical information system projects: insights from two cross-sectional surveys', *Implementation Science* 6, 15, www.implementationscience.com/content/6/1/15.

Parish C (2012) 'Creating the right conditions for person-centred care to flourish', *Learning Disability Practice* 15, 9, 6–8.

Parkin P (2009) *Managing Change in Healthcare Using Action Research* (London: Sage).

Parlour R and McCormack B (2012) 'Blending critical realist and emancipatory practice development methodologies: making critical realism work in nursing research', *Nursing Inquiry* 19, 4, 308–21.

Paton RA and McCalman J (2008) *Change Management: A Guide to Effective Implementation* (3rd edn). (London: Sage).

Pawson R and Tilley N (1997) *Realistic Evaluation* (London: Sage).

Pedersen LM, Nielsen KJ and Kines P (2012) 'Realistic evaluation as a new way to design and evaluate occupational safety interventions', *Safety Science* 50, 1, 48–54.

Peek C, Higgins I, Milson-Hawke S, McMillan M and Harper D (2007) 'Towards innovation: the development of a person-centered model of care for older people in the acute setting', *Contemporary Nurse* 26, 2, 164–76.

Perron A, Rudge T and Holmes D (2010) 'Citizen minds, citizen bodies: the citizenship experience and the government of mentally ill persons', *Nursing Philosophy* 11, 100–11.

Pittam G, Boyce M, Secker J, Lockett H and Samele C (2010) 'Employment advice in primary care: a realistic evaluation', *Health and Social Care in the Community* 18, 6, 598–606.

Pommier J, Guével M-R and Jourdan D (2010) 'Evaluation of health promotion in schools: a realistic evaluation approach using mixed methods', *BMC Public Health* 10, 43 doi:10.1186/1471-2458-10-43.

Porter S and O'Halloran P (2012) 'The use and limitation of realistic evaluation as a tool for evidence-based practice: a critical realist perspective', *Nursing Inquiry* 19, 1, 18–28.

Price B (2008) 'Strategies to help nurses cope with change in the healthcare setting', *Nursing Standard* 22, 48, 50–6.

Price B (2010) 'Disseminating best practice through publication in journals', *Nursing Standard* 24, 26, 35–41.

Prochaska JO and DiClemente CC (1992) 'Stages of change in the modification of problem behaviours', *Progress in Behaviour Modification* 28, 183–218.

Qian Y and Daniels TD (2008) 'A communication model of employee cynicism toward organizational change', *Corporate Communications* 13, 3, 319–32.

Quatro SA, Waldman DA and Galvin BM (2007) 'Developing holistic leaders: four domains for leadership development and practice', *Human Resource Management Review* 17, 4, 427–41.

RCN (Royal College of Nursing) (2009) *Measuring for Quality in Health and Social Care: An RCN Position Statement*, http://tinyurl.com/6c6s3gd, accessed 14/3/14.

RCN/RCP (Royal College of Nursing/Royal College of Physicians) (2006) *Acute and Multidisciplinary Working: Policy Statement 16/2006* (London: RCN/RCP).

Reed J and Turner J (2005) 'Appreciating change in cancer services: an evaluation of service development strategies', *Journal of Health Organization and Management* 19, 2, 163–76.

Regan P (2011) 'Critical issues in practice development: localism and public health reforms', *Community Practitioner* 84, 3, 32–5.

Reid G, Kneafsey R, Long A, Hulme C and Wright H (2007) 'Change and transformation: the impact of an action-research evaluation on the development of a new service', *Learning in Health and Social Care* 6, 2, 61–71.

Reinhardt AC and Keller T (2009) 'Implementing interdisciplinary practice change in an international health-care organization', *International Journal of Nursing Practice* 15, 4, 318–25.

Richens Y, Rycroft-Malone J and Morrell C (2004) 'Getting guidelines into practice: a literature review', *Nursing Standard* 18, 50, 33–40.

Rieg LS, Mason CH and Preston K (2006) 'Spiritual care: practical guidelines for rehabilitation nurses', *Rehabilitation Nursing* 31, 6, 249–56.

Rise MB, Solbjør M, Lara MC, Westerlund H, Grimstad H et al. (2013) 'Same description, different values: how service users and providers define patient and public involvement in health care', *Health Expectations* 16, 3, 266–76.

Roberts P and Priest H (2006) 'Reliability and validity in research', *Nursing Standard* 20, 44, 41–5.

Rodgers M, Sowden A, Petticrew M, Arai L, Roberts H et al. (2009) 'Testing methodological guidance on the conduct of narrative synthesis in systematic reviews', *Evaluation* 15, 1, 47–71.

Rogers EM (1995) *Diffusion of Innovations* (4th edn). (New York: Free Press).

Rose D, Fleischmann P and Schofield P (2010) 'Perceptions of user involvement: a user-led study', *The International Journal of Social Psychiatry* 56, 4, 389–401.

Rowlands I, Nicholas D, Russell B, Canty N and Watkinson A (2011) 'Social media use in the research workflow', *Learned Publishing* 24, 183–95.

Rycroft-Malone J, Fontenla M, Bick D and Seers K (2010) 'A realistic evaluation: the case of protocol-based care', *Implementation Science* 5, 38 doi:10.1186/1748-5908-5-38.

Rycroft-Malone J, Dopson S, Degner L, Hutchinson AM, Morgan D et al. (2009) 'Study protocol for the translating research in elder care (TREC): building context through case studies in long-term care project (project two)', *Implementation Science* 4, 53.

Rycroft-Malone J, Wilkinson JE, Burton CR, Andrews G, Ariss S et al. (2011) 'Implementing health research through academic and clinical partnerships: a realistic evaluation of the Collaborations for Leadership in Applied Health Research and Care (CLAHRC)', *Implementation Science* 6, 74 doi:10.1186/1748-5908-6-74.

Sandelowski M, Voils CI, Leeman J and Crandell JL (2012) 'Mapping the mixed methods-mixed research synthesis terrain', *Journal of Mixed Methods Research* 6, 4, 317–31.

Sanders K, Odell J and Webster J (2013) 'Learning to be a practice developer', pp. 18–44, in McCormack B, Manley K and Titchen A (eds) *Practice Development in Nursing and Healthcare* (2nd edn). (Chichester: Wiley Blackwell).

Schifalacqua M, Costello C and Denman W (2009) 'Roadmap for planned change. Part 1. Change leadership and project management', *Nurse Leader* 7, 6, 26–9.

Scott T, Mannion R, Davies HTO and Marshall MN (2003) 'Implementing culture change in health care: theory and practice', *International Journal of Quality in Healthcare* 15, 2, 111–18.

Scottish Government (2009) *The Health-Care Quality Strategy for Scotland* (Edinburgh: Scottish Government).

Shaw T (2013) 'Approaches to practice development', pp. 66–87, in McCormack B, Manley K and Garbett R (eds) *Practice Development in Nursing* (Chichester: Wiley-Blackwell).

Sheehan N and Hayles J (2006) 'Facing up to the challenges of the practice development unit: a leader's perspective', *Practice Development in Health Care* 5, 1, 20–5.

Skinner D (2004) 'Evaluation and change management: rhetoric and reality', *Human Resources Management Journal* 14, 3, 5–19.

Smith E, Ross F, Donovan S, Manthorpe J, Brearley S et al. (2008) 'Service user involvement in nursing, midwifery and health visiting research: a review of evidence and practice', *International Journal of Nursing Studies* 45, 2, 298–315.

State Government of Victoria (2012) *Best Care for Older People Everywhere: The Toolkit 2012* (Melbourne: State Government of Victoria).

Surakka T (2008) 'The nurse manager's work in the hospital environment during the 1990s and 2000s: responsibility, accountability and expertise in nursing leadership', *Journal of Nursing Management* 16, 5, 525–34.

Tashakkori A and Teddlie C (2003) *Handbook of Mixed Methods in Social and Behavioral Research* (Thousand Oaks, CA: Sage).

Thompson DR, Chau JPC and Lopez V (2006) 'Barriers to, and facilitators of, research utilisation: a survey of Hong Kong registered nurses', *International Journal of Evidence Based Healthcare* 4, 2, 77–82.

Thornton L (2011) 'Person-centred dementia: an essential component of ethical nursing care', *Canadian Nursing Home* 22, 3, 10–14.

Timmins P and Miller C (2007) 'Making evaluations realistic: the challenge of complexity', *Support for Learning* 22, 1, 9–16.

Titchen A and McMahon (2013) 'Practice development as radical gardening: enabling creativity and innovation', pp. 212–32, in McCormack B, Manley K and Titchen A (eds) *Practice Development in Nursing and Healthcare* (2nd edn). (Chichester: Wiley-Blackwell).

Titchen A, Dewing J and Manley K (2013) 'Getting going with facilitation skills in practice development', pp. 109–29, in McCormack B, Manley K and Titchen A (eds) *Practice Development in Nursing and Healthcare* (2nd edn). (Chichester: Wiley-Blackwell).

Tolson D and Schofield I (2012) 'Football reminiscence for men with dementia: lessons from a realistic evaluation', *Nursing Inquiry* 19, 1, 63–70.

Tong A, Lopez-Vargas P, Howell M, Phoon R, Johnson D et al. (2012) 'Consumer involvement in topic and outcome selection in the development of clinical practice guidelines', *Health Expectations* 15, 4, 410–23.

Tritter JQ (2009) 'Revolution or evolution: the challenges of conceptualizing patient and public involvement in a consumerist world', *Health Expectations* 12, 3, 275–87.

TwoCan Associates (2011) *Evaluation of the 'User Involvement in Local Diabetes Care' Project* (London: Diabetes UK).

Van den Pol-Grevelink A, Jukema JS and Smits CHM (2012) 'Person-centred care and job satisfaction of caregivers in nursing homes: a systematic review of the impact of different forms of person-centred care on various dimensions of job satisfaction', *International Journal of Geriatric Psychiatry* 27, 3, 219–29.

Van der Zijpp TJ and Dowling J (2009) 'A case study of learning to become a PD facilitator: "Climbing the tree"', *Practice Development in Health Care* 8, 4, 200–15.

Virani T, Lemieux-Charles L, Davis DA and Berta W (2009) 'Sustaining change. Once evidence based practices are transferred: what then?', *Healthcare Quarterly* 12, 1, 89–96.

Wade DT (2005) 'Ethics, audit and research: all shades of grey', *British Medical Journal* 330, 7489, 468–71.

Walsh K, Jordan Z and Appolloni L (2009) 'The problematic art of conversation: communication and health practice evolution', *Practice Development in Health Care* 8, 3, 166–79.

Walsh KD, Crisp J and Moss C (2011) 'Psychodynamic perspectives on organizational change and their relevance to transformational practice development', *International Journal of Nursing Practice* 17, 205–12.

Walumbwa FO, Wang P, Wang H, Schaubroeck J and Avolio BJ (2010) 'Psychological processes linking authentic leadership to follower behaviors', *The Leadership Quarterly* 21, 5, 901–14.

Wand T, White K and Patching J (2011) 'Realistic evaluation of an emergency department-based mental health nurse practitioner outpatient service in Australia', *Nursing and Health Sciences* 13, 2, 199–206.

Ward J, de Motte C and Bailey D (2013) 'Service user involvement in the evaluation of psycho-social intervention for self-harm: a systematic literature review', *Journal of Research in Nursing* 18, 2, 114–30.

Weiner BJ, Amick H and Lee SY (2008) 'Review: conceptualization and measurement of organizational readiness for change: a review of the literature in health services research and other fields', *Medical Care Research and Review* 65, 4, 379–436.

Welch R and McCarville RE (2003) 'Discovering conditions for staff acceptance of organizational change', *Journal of Park and Recreation Administration* 21, 2, 22–43.

Welford C (2006) 'Change management and quality', *Nursing Management* 13, 5, 23–6.

White C (2005) 'My development as a PDU leader: leadership and power', *Practice Development in Health Care* 4, 4, 225–30.

Wiley J, Westbrook M, Greenfield JR, Day RO and Braithwaite J (2014) 'Shared decision-making: the perspectives of young adults with type 1 diabetes mellitus', *Patient Preference and Adherence* 8, 423–35.

Wilson V and McCormack B (2006) 'Critical realism as emancipatory action: the case for realistic evaluation in practice development', *Nursing Philosophy* 7, 1, 45–57.

Wilson V, McCormack B and Ives G (2006) 'Re-generating the "self " in learning : developing a culture of supportive learning in practice', *Learning in Health and Social Care* 5, 2, 90–105.

Windish DM and Diener-West M (2006) 'A clinician-educator's roadmap to choosing and interpreting statistical tests', *Journal of General Internal Medicine* 21, 6, 656–60.

Wong CA and Cummings GG (2009) 'The influence of authentic leadership behaviors on trust and work outcomes of health care staff', *Journal of Leadership Studies* 3, 2, 6–23.

Wright S (2010) 'Dealing with resistance', *Nursing Standard* 24, 23, 18–20.

Index